Herbal Solutions for Viral Challenges

A Journey Through Herbal Antiviral Practices

Sarah Emerson

Table of Contents

INTRODUCTION **6**

CHAPTER I. Understanding Viral Challenges **8**

What Are Viruses? 8

Common Viral Infections and Their Impact.................. 11

The Evolution of Viral Threats 13

Challenges in Conventional Treatments 16

CHAPTER II. Exploring Herbal Medicine **20**

History and Tradition of Herbal Medicine 20

Key Components of Herbal Remedies 23

Herbal Medicine and Modern Healthcare 26

CHAPTER III. Building Your Herbal Toolkit **29**

Identifying and Sourcing Herbs 29

Basic Principles of Herbal Preparation 31

Herbal Formulations and Combinations 34

Safety Guidelines and Precautions 37

CHAPTER IV. Herbal Solutions for Specific Viral Infections **41**

Influenza and Common Cold 41

Herpes Viruses 44

Respiratory Syncytial Virus (RSV) 47

Human Immunodeficiency Virus (HIV) 51

Hepatitis Viruses 54

Emerging Viral Threats (e.g., Zika, Ebola) 57

CHAPTER V. Integrating Herbal Practices into Daily Life . 61

Herbal Immune Support 61

Herbal Remedies for Prevention 64

Herbal Treatments for Acute Infections 67

Long-term Management Strategies 70

CHAPTER VI. Case Studies and Success Stories 73

Personal Experiences with Herbal Antiviral Practices ... 73

Testimonials from Practitioners and Patients 75

Real-life Applications of Herbal Solutions 78

CHAPTER VII. Herbal Medicine and Holistic Health 81

The Mind-Body Connection in Healing 81

Herbal Practices for Emotional Well-being 83

Lifestyle Factors and Herbal Support 86

Herbal Medicine as Part of a Comprehensive Health Plan
.... 89

CHAPTER VIII. Overcoming Challenges and Resistance ... 92

Addressing Skepticism and Misconceptions 92

Navigating Legal and Regulatory Hurdles 95

Overcoming Cultural and Societal Barriers 97

Future Directions and Opportunities 100

**CHAPTER IX. Herbal Remedies in Traditional Medicine
Systems 103**

Ayurveda and Herbal Antiviral Practices 103

Traditional Chinese Medicine (TCM) Approaches 105

Indigenous Herbal Healing Practices 109

Integrating Global Herbal Traditions 112

CHAPTER X. Herbal Medicine and Public Health 115

Role of Herbal Medicine in Pandemic Preparedness .. 115

Community-Based Herbal Healthcare Initiatives 118

Herbal Medicine in Resource-limited Settings 121

CONCLUSION 125

INTRODUCTION

The thorough study "Herbal Solutions for Viral Challenges: A Journey Through Herbal Antiviral Practices" delves into the relationship between herbal therapy and fighting viral infections. The advent and dissemination of viral infections provide severe obstacles to public health systems and individual well-being in today's global environment. In this context, herbal medicines, with their historical value and current applicability, emerge as practical means of countering viral threats.

This book thoroughly explores the science, history, and practical applications of herbal antiviral practices as it digs into the diverse web of herbal traditions from around the globe. It aims to close the knowledge gap between conventional wisdom and modern medical practices by giving readers a comprehensive grasp of the ways in which medicinal plants can be used to control, prevent, and treat viral infections.

Readers will learn about the complex mechanics behind viral infections, the historical evolution of viral threats, and the difficulties associated with traditional treatment approaches through an experience- and expertise-driven trip. After that, the book explores the background and customs of herbal medicine, revealing the tried-and-true cures that have been inherited down the ages. It delves into the science underlying the antiviral qualities of herbal remedies, clarifying the bioactive ingredients and modes of action that make some plants formidable opponents of viruses.

In addition, readers will discover the essential elements of herbal treatments and gain knowledge on how to recognize, obtain, and process medicinal plants for optimal effectiveness and safety. The book also explores the use of herbal medicine in contemporary healthcare, looking at how it fits into established treatment plans and how it might strengthen and supplement current therapeutic modalities.

Upon commencing this voyage through herbal antiviral techniques, readers will come across an abundance of knowledge, perspectives, and helpful advice to enable them in their personal pursuits of health and well-being.

With the ability to navigate viral problems through herbal medicine's power, this book is a reliable companion and resource for anybody looking for prevention measures, supportive care, or alternative therapies.

CHAPTER I

Understanding Viral Challenges

What Are Viruses?

Viruses are a fantastic class of biological objects that exist on the brink between existence and inanimate matter. In contrast to bacteria, fungi, plants, and animals, viruses do not have the cellular components required for self-sufficient existence. They lack organelles, a cellular structure, and metabolic functions, making them acellular. On the other hand, viruses have genetic material (DNA or RNA) that contains the instructions needed for their propagation and reproduction. The capsid, a protein coat that encases the genetic material, serves as both a protective barrier and a means of facilitating the virus's interactions with host cells. In order to help them infect cells and elude the host's immune response, many viruses also possess an outer lipid envelope made from the membrane of the host cell.

A virus's lifecycle starts when it comes into contact with a vulnerable host cell. Viruses target distinct cell types inside their host organism and are very precise in whom they choose to infect. The initial stage of a viral infection typically involves the virus attaching itself to particular receptors on the outermost layer of the host cell. This attachment sets off a chain of events that eventually leads to the virus entering the host cell, frequently through endocytosis or fusion with the cell membrane. The virus distributes its genetic material into the host cell, where it uses the biological machinery to duplicate its genome and make viral proteins. New virus particles are created from the newly produced viral components, and these particles have the ability to infect additional cells and disseminate the infection throughout the entire body.

The remarkable ability of viruses to change and adapt over time presents a considerable barrier to efforts focused on managing and treating viral illnesses. During the course of viral replication, mutations may occur naturally or as a result of the host immune system's or antiviral medications' selection pressures. The structure and functionality of viral proteins can be changed by these mutations, which can impact the virus's capacity to infect cells, elude the immune system, or react to antiviral medications. A selection advantage may occasionally be conferred by mutations, making it possible for the virus to multiply more effectively or spread more quickly within a host population. This feature is especially noticeable in RNA viruses with rapid mutation rates, such as influenza and HIV, which exist as different quasispecies or groups of closely related varieties.

Viral transmission can happen through a number of channels, such as insect vectors, infected food or water, body fluids, and respiratory droplets. Viruses can spread quickly among populations once they've been introduced to a new host, resulting in outbreaks and epidemics. Certain viruses can spread from animals to people due to their zoonotic origins, which makes them a continual concern for the emergence of infectious diseases. The new coronavirus SARS-CoV-2 that produced the COVID-19 pandemic is a sobering reminder of the catastrophic effects that zoonotic viruses can have on economies and public health around the world.

Viruses are known to cause illness and destruction, yet they are also crucial to ecosystems and evolutionary processes. They use predation and cell-to-cell genetic material transfer to affect the diversity and abundance of their host organisms. By encouraging the selection of beneficial features or promoting genetic exchange through mechanisms like horizontal gene transfer, viruses can influence the evolution of host populations. Furthermore, viruses play a role in the dynamics of ecosystems and the cycle of nutrients by interacting intimately with their hosts.

Viruses offer opportunities as well as difficulties to the medical community. Numerous lives have been saved, and the global burden of disease has decreased as a result of the development of vaccinations and antiviral medications, which have significantly advanced the prevention and treatment of viral diseases. Nonetheless, the necessity for ongoing virology research and innovation is highlighted by the rise of drug-resistant viral strains and the persistent threat of new and reemerging infectious illnesses.

In order to prevent viral infections and lessen their adverse effects on human as well as animal health, it is imperative to comprehend the nature of viruses. This covers both basic research to clarify the molecular underpinnings of viral disease and replication and applied research to provide novel vaccines, treatments, and diagnostic instruments. Furthermore, early epidemic detection and containment depend heavily on efforts to monitor and survey virus populations in both human and animal populations.

To sum up, viruses are unique organisms that are difficult to categorize within the biological order. Their distinct characteristics enable them to flourish in many settings and engage in interactions with a wide variety of host organisms. Certain viruses contribute to the diversity of life on Earth and cause sickness and misery, whereas other viruses are beneficial to ecosystems. Scientists can learn about fundamental biological processes and create plans to stop and manage viral infections by researching viruses and how they interact with their host organisms.

Common Viral Infections and Their Impact

Every year, millions of people worldwide suffer from common viral infections, which have a substantial negative impact on public health due to increased morbidity, mortality, and financial expenses. Numerous different viruses that target different human organ systems and tissues are the source of these infections. The common cold, influenza, and also respiratory syncytial virus (RSV) are among the most frequent viral illnesses that impact the respiratory system. Common cold symptoms include runny nose, cough, sore throat, and nasal congestion. The common cold is mainly caused by rhinoviruses. The common cold is usually mild and self-limiting. However, it can still be uncomfortable and inconvenient, especially for vulnerable groups, including small children, the elderly, and people with underlying medical disorders. Influenza is a more dangerous respiratory virus that can cause severe illness, hospitalization, and even death, particularly in high-risk individuals. Influenza viruses cause influenza. Seasonal influenza outbreaks cause considerable illness and mortality each year in many parts of the world, underscoring the significance of immunization and public health initiatives to stop transmission.

Respiratory syncytial virus (RSV) is another common viral infection that affects the respiratory system, particularly in young children. RSV infections can cause anything from minor cold-like symptoms to severe lower respiratory tract infections that need to be treated in a hospital or intensive care unit, like pneumonia and bronchiolitis. RSV is a significant contributor to hospital admissions and healthcare costs annually, as it is the primary cause of respiratory diseases in newborns and early children. The fact that there is presently no authorized vaccination for RSV despite decades of study emphasizes the necessity of ongoing efforts to develop therapeutic and preventive measures.

Virus-related gastroenteritis, in addition to respiratory infections, is a significant public health concern, especially in low-resource environments and among susceptible groups like young children, the elderly, and immunocompromised individuals. Noroviruses, rotaviruses, and enteric adenoviruses are the most prevalent viruses that cause viral gastroenteritis. They are highly contagious and can also spread through contaminated food, water, and surfaces. Typical symptoms of viral gastroenteritis include fever, vomiting, diarrhea, and abdominal pain. In more severe cases, these symptoms can result in electrolyte imbalances and dehydration. While the majority of viral gastroenteritis episodes are self-limiting and go away in a few days, more severe infections might need to be treated with supportive care and rehydration therapy.

Sexually transmitted infections (STIs), such as the human papillomavirus (HPV), herpes simplex virus (HSV), and human immunodeficiency virus (HIV), are another category of prevalent viral illnesses. With several strains causing different clinical manifestations, such as genital warts and cervical, anal, and oropharyngeal malignancies, HPV is the most common sexually transmitted infection (STI) in the world. The importance of vaccination programs as a public health intervention is highlighted by the fact that vaccination against HPV has been demonstrated to be very successful in preventing infection and lowering the incidence of disorders connected to HPV.

Herpes Simplex virus (HSV) infections are also frequent; HSV-1 is primarily responsible for oral herpes, often known as cold sores, while HSV-2 is the cause of genital herpes. Even while HSV infections are usually minor and self-limiting, susceptible persons may experience severe discomfort and stigma if outbreaks occur frequently. At now, there is no known treatment for HSV infection;

however, antiviral drugs can help manage symptoms and also lessen the frequency and severity of outbreaks.

Thirty-eight million people are thought to be infected with HIV/AIDS worldwide, making it a serious global health concern. HIV can spread through intercourse, blood-to-blood contact, and mother-to-child transmission during pregnancy, childbirth, and nursing. In the absence of medical intervention, HIV infection develops into acquired immunodeficiency syndrome (AIDS), a disorder marked by a weakened immune system and heightened vulnerability to opportunistic infections and cancers. But because of developments in antiretroviral therapy (ART), HIV infection is no longer a death sentence for many people—instead, it's now a chronic, treatable illness. Achieving viral suppression, enhancing immunological function, and lowering the risk of transmission to others need early diagnosis, timely ART therapy, and adherence to treatment.

In summary, widespread viral infections pose a serious threat to global public health, affecting people of all ages and socioeconomic status. These infections can result in a broad spectrum of symptoms and side effects, ranging from little discomfort to severe disease and even death. In order to lower the incidence of viral infections and safeguard people's health, prevention measures such as immunization, safe sexual behavior, hand cleanliness, and public health campaigns are essential. Furthermore, in order to create efficient plans for managing and controlling viral infections in the future, further study into the epidemiology, pathophysiology, and therapy of these illnesses is necessary.

The Evolution of Viral Threats

Viral dangers have evolved through a complex and dynamic process, including genetic, ecological, and socioeconomic elements. Viruses are ancient creatures that have spent millions of years co-evolving with their hosts. They are constantly diversifying and adapting to take advantage of new ecological niches and outwit host defenses. Novel viral infections capable of triggering epidemics and pandemics with severe effects on human health and civilization have emerged as a result of this continuing evolutionary arms race.

Genetic diversity is one of the leading forces that contribute to the evolution of viruses. Because their replication machinery is prone to errors and does not have methods for proofreading the viral genome, viruses have high rates of mutation. Thus, viruses give rise to a variety of closely related populations of variants known as quasispecies, which can evolve quickly in response to selection pressures like host immunity or antiviral therapies. Because of their high rates of mutation and genetic variety, RNA viruses, in particular, are more likely to give rise to novel strains that have increased virulence, transmissibility, or resistance to antiviral medications.

Another essential aspect impacting the evolution of viral risks is the expansion of host ranges. The capacity of many viruses to switch between multiple host species is referred to as cross-species transmission or spillover. Animal-borne zoonotic viruses are a continual danger to human health, as they can cause infectious diseases. Deforestation, urbanization, intensification of agriculture, and the commerce of wildlife can all lead to an increase in the frequency of human-animal contact, which in turn can facilitate the spread of zoonotic viruses from wildlife reservoirs to human populations. The Ebola virus, which is thought to spread to humans through contact with sick animals like fruit bats, and avian influenza viruses, which can spread from birds to humans through intimate contact with infected poultry, are two examples of zoonotic viruses.

The evolution of viral risks is significantly shaped by environmental variables as well. A number of viral infections are transmitted by vector species like ticks and mosquitoes, whose range and abundance can be altered by climate change, habitat degradation, and ecosystem disruption. The geographic distribution of vector-borne diseases can be influenced by changes in land use, temperature, and rainfall patterns. This can result in the resurgence of formerly endemic diseases as well as the formation of new infectious hotspots. For instance, urbanization, population increase, and climate change have all been connected to the spread of dengue fever, a virus carried by mosquitoes that infect humans. These factors facilitate the growth of mosquito vectors and the virus's dissemination.

Viral dangers evolve in part due to human behavior and socioeconomic variables. Travel, trade, and globalization all contribute to the quick cross-border transmission of infectious diseases, which gives viruses a chance to invade new areas and prey on vulnerable populations. Urbanization, poverty, and population development can lead to unsanitary circumstances, overcrowding, and inadequate healthcare infrastructure, all of which raise the possibility of viral transmission and the intensity of outbreaks. Wet markets, bushmeat hunting, and traditional healing practices are examples of sociocultural practices that highlight the link between human and animal health and may contribute to the transmission of zoonotic illnesses from animals to humans.

The development of viral risks poses significant obstacles to activities aimed at controlling disease and promoting public health. Identification of newly emerging viral infections and prompt implementation of treatments to prevent or minimize outbreaks depend on rapid detection, surveillance, and reaction. Public health education, vector control, and vaccination are some of the strategies that can help stop the spread of viral illnesses and safeguard vulnerable groups. Research and innovation expenditures are also necessary to provide novel vaccines, treatments, and diagnostic tools to combat resurgent and emerging viral threats.

In conclusion, genetic variety, host range extension, environmental changes, and human behavior all play essential roles in the complex and multidimensional evolution of viral hazards. Reducing the impact of infectious illnesses on society and human health requires an understanding of the mechanisms influencing the genesis and spread of viral viruses. Through the implementation of a One Health strategy that acknowledges the interdependence of environmental, animal, and human health, we may more effectively anticipate and address the changing obstacles presented by viral threats in the twenty-first century.

Challenges in Conventional Treatments

The peculiarities of viruses and the constraints of available therapeutic choices present difficulties in the routine treatment of viral infections. In contrast to bacteria, which are living things with unique cellular compositions and metabolic activities, viruses are acellular substances that reproduce only in their host cells. It is challenging to create medications that selectively target viruses without endangering host cells because of this fundamental distinction. Furthermore, viruses are genetically variable and have high rates of mutation, which enable them to develop resistance to antiviral medications swiftly. Because of this, many traditional antiviral drugs have a limited therapeutic window and may eventually lose their effectiveness due to viral strain resistance.

The limited range of action of many antiviral medications is another difficulty for traditional therapies for viral infections. The majority of antiviral drugs are ineffective against unrelated infections because they only target particular viruses or viral families. Due to this restriction, patients may exhibit viral infection symptoms in clinical settings without a conclusive diagnosis of the underlying cause. In these situations, broad-spectrum antiviral medications that target several viruses may be used empirically, but in comparison to targeted therapy, these drugs may be less successful or have a higher risk of side effects.

Another factor to take into account when using traditional antiviral medications is the mode of administration. Many antiviral drugs must be taken orally or intravenously, which can be difficult or uncomfortable for certain patients, especially those with viral infections that are mild or self-limiting. Furthermore, a number of variables that differ from person to person and impact treatment outcomes, including drug absorption, distribution, metabolism, and excretion, can impact how effective antiviral medications are. Specific antiviral drugs, for instance, may not be well absorbed via the mouth or may need to be taken at different doses in those with compromised liver or kidney function.

Another area for improvement in the treatment of viral infections is drug adherence. Strict adherence to dose regimens is necessary for many antiviral drugs in order to achieve therapeutic efficacy and avoid the emergence of drug resistance. Adherence to therapy, however, may be impacted by variables such as drug costs, side effects, complicated dosage schedules, and patient education. The management of viral infections, especially chronic or recurrent illnesses, can be complicated by non-adherence to antiviral therapy, which can result in treatment failure, return of symptoms, and the establishment of drug-resistant virus strains.

Apart from these difficulties, the creation of novel antiviral medications encounters impediments like protracted and expensive procedures for drug research and development, regulatory mandates, and market dynamics. In contrast to other therapeutic categories like antibacterial agents, the pipeline for new antiviral treatments is still somewhat small despite advancements in molecular virology and drug development technologies. Pharmacies looking to engage in antiviral drug research have difficulties due to the high failure rate of drug ideas in preclinical and clinical trials, as well as the unpredictability of market demand and competition from generic drugs.

Moreover, managing viral infections is significantly hampered by the development of viral resistance to current antiviral medications. Viral genome mutations that provide lower susceptibility to therapeutic action, as well as changes in viral replication or entrance pathways that circumvent the drug's inhibitory effects, are some of the processes by which viruses might develop resistance to antiviral drugs. The emergence of drug-resistant virus strains has the potential to compromise the efficacy of antiviral therapy and pose challenges for medical professionals in making treatment decisions.

The problems with traditional viral infection therapies must be addressed with a multifaceted strategy that incorporates developments in drug discovery technology, clinical practice recommendations, and molecular virology. Understanding the molecular mechanisms underlying drug resistance, pathogenicity, and viral replication is crucial for discovering new targets for antiviral therapy and creating innovative therapeutic approaches. To effectively manage viral infections and lessen their adverse effects on society and human health, it is also essential to implement programs that enhance patient education, healthcare access, and public health infrastructure. Through cooperative efforts, scholars, medical professionals, legislators, and business partners can enhance the effectiveness, security, and availability of antiviral therapies for viral illnesses.

CHAPTER II

Exploring Herbal Medicine

History and Tradition of Herbal Medicine

Herbal medicine has a long history that spans thousands of years and is practiced in many cultures and civilizations worldwide. Phytotherapy, botanical medicine, and herbal medicine are terms used to describe the use of plants and plant extracts for therapeutic purposes. Herbal medicine has been used for at least 60,000 years; archeological findings indicate that humans have been using plants for therapeutic purposes for much longer than is known in written history. Sophisticated systems of herbal medicine were developed by early civilizations like the Sumerians, Egyptians, Chinese, and Greeks. These systems were founded on trial and error, accumulated knowledge passed down through generations, and empirical observation. For instance, medicinal plants were employed to cure a variety of illnesses in ancient Egypt. Medical texts such as the Ebers Papyrus, which was written around 1550 BCE, mention herbal remedies. Herbal formulations are essential for reestablishing harmony and balance in the body, and traditional Chinese medicine (TCM) has a long history of using them in its holistic approach to health as well as wellness.

Herbal medicine has been utilized historically by shamans, medicine men, healers, and wise women who were knowledgeable about the therapeutic uses of many plants. Herbal medicine reflects a holistic view of health that includes the physical, mental, emotional, and also spiritual aspects of well-being and is intricately entwined with spiritual beliefs, cultural traditions, and rituals in many indigenous societies. Indigenous healing practices place a strong emphasis on the relationship between people and the natural world and acknowledge that plants have healing properties of their own and should be treated as sacred gifts from the planet.

Herbal medicine flourished in Europe during the Middle Ages as monastic communities conserved and developed the herbal knowledge passed down from past civilizations. Herbal medicine originated in monasteries, where monks grew medicinal gardens, translated old manuscripts, and created herbal cures for a range of ailments. The development of herbal medicine in Europe was aided by the significant contributions of individuals like the German herbalist and abbess Hildegard of Bingen in the 12th century. Even now, practitioners of herbal medicine are still motivated by Hildegard's writings about the therapeutic qualities of plants and her all-encompassing approach to healing.

The translation and distribution of classical writings from ancient Greece and Rome contributed to the Renaissance's renewal of interest in herbal therapy. In England, herbalists like John Gerard and Nicholas Culpeper wrote large herbals that described the botanical traits, therapeutic applications, and uses of various plants. These herbals offered significant insights into the pharmacological effects of medicinal plants and their applications in clinical practice, making them essential resources for doctors, apothecaries, and herbalists.

Herbal medicine saw a drop in popularity in many parts of the world in the 19th and also 20th centuries as pharmaceutical medications and synthetic substances replaced it as the primary means of treating illnesses. However, a newfound appreciation for the therapeutic potential of natural treatments and growing worries about the side effects, cost, and accessibility of conventional medications drove a resurgence of interest in herbal medicine in the late 20th and early 21st centuries.

With millions of people using herbal medicines for preventive, supportive, and curative purposes in their healthcare routines, herbal therapy is becoming a significant part of complementary and alternative medicine (CAM) practices worldwide. Widely accessible over-the-counter and online, herbal supplements, teas, tinctures, and topical therapies are promoted for a range of medical issues, from mild illnesses to chronic disorders. Herbal medicine is also still used in traditional medical systems like indigenous medicine, TCM, and Ayurveda, where it is ingrained in spiritual beliefs, communal customs, and cultural traditions.

Herbal medicine has a long history and is widely used, but it has difficulties in the current healthcare environment, such as problems with quality control, safety, efficacy, and legislation. The diverse range of herbal products' composition and potency, coupled with the possibility of contamination, adulteration, and mislabeling, emphasizes the necessity of implementing standardized production procedures, quality assurance systems, and regulatory supervision. Concerns regarding adverse effects, contraindications, and herb-drug interactions further emphasize how crucial it is for patients and healthcare professionals to work together to make educated decisions when including herbal treatments in treatment plans.

Notwithstanding these difficulties, the history and practice of herbal medicine continue to stand as evidence of the continuing partnership between people and plants in the search for well-being. Herbal medicine continues to be an invaluable and adaptable tool for fostering well-being, encouraging self-care, and improving the quality of life for people and communities worldwide as interest in holistic and integrative approaches to healthcare grows. Herbal medicine has the potential to play a significant part in the healthcare systems of the future by adopting scientific rigor and evidence-based principles while still

acknowledgin   the wisdom of   ancient   therapeutic
g techniques.

Key Components of Herbal Remedies

The complex processes by which plant chemicals have antiviral actions against a variety of viral infections are explored in the science behind the antiviral characteristics of herbal remedies. Phytochemicals are a broad class of chemical molecules that have evolved by plants to perform a variety of defense-related tasks against environmental stresses, diseases, and predators. Numerous of these phytochemicals have antiviral solid properties that affect various phases of the viral life cycle and obstruct viral assembly, replication, or penetration into host cells. Polyphenols, a family of phytochemicals having antiviral qualities that include flavonoids, phenolic acids, and tannins found in fruits, vegetables, herbs, and spices, are among the most researched groups of phytochemicals. A wide range of RNA and DNA viruses, such as the respiratory syncytial virus (RSV), herpes simplex, influenza, and human immunodeficiency virus (HIV), are susceptible to the antiviral effects of polyphenols.

For their antiviral qualities, flavonoids like kaempferol, quercetin, and epigallocatechin gallate (EGCG) have been investigated the most among polyphenols. Viral reproduction has been demonstrated to be inhibited by these substances through inhibiting viral enzymes, obstructing the attachment and also the entry of viruses into host cells, or modifying the host immune system's reaction to viral infection. For instance, it has been discovered that quercetin inhibits the replication of respiratory viruses, including RSV and influenza A virus, by preventing viral polymerase activity and lowering the synthesis of pro inflammatory cytokines that aid in the pathogenesis of the virus.

Intense antiviral action is also shown by phenolic acids, such as rosmarinic acid and caffeic acid, against a range of viral infections. These substances work against viruses by interfering with the production of viral proteins, preventing the virus from attaching itself to host cells or adjusting the host's immune system in reaction to a viral infection. For example, it has been demonstrated that rosmarinic acid, which is present in herbs like rosemary and lemon balm, inhibits the replication of the herpes simplex virus (HSV) and the human cytomegalovirus (HCMV) by interfering with the replication of viral DNA and early gene expression.

Researchers have looked at the antiviral capabilities of tannins, a different family of polyphenols, against enveloped viruses, including HIV and influenza. Tannins are believed to work against viruses by attaching to their envelope proteins and obstructing the virus's ability to enter host cells. This stops viruses from infecting and multiplying. For instance, it has been demonstrated that ellagitannins, which are present in pomegranate extract, prevent the influenza virus from attaching to and fusing with cellular membranes, preventing the virus from infecting host cells.

Alkaloids, terpenoids, and essential oils are other types of phytochemicals with antiviral qualities in addition to polyphenols. It has been demonstrated that alkaloids, such as berberine and sanguinarine, which are present in bloodroot and goldenseal, have antiviral properties against a range of RNA and DNA viruses, such as the hepatitis B virus (HBV), herpes simplex, and influenza. These substances target viral enzymes or obstruct the creation of viral proteins to obstruct viral replication. Terpenoids like the thymol and carvacrol found in the essential oils of oregano and also thyme have antiviral properties against respiratory viruses like the rhinovirus and influenza by rupturing the integrity of the viral membrane and blocking viral multiplication. The antiviral qualities of essential oils derived from plants like peppermint, eucalyptus, and tea tree have also been studied; certain oils have demonstrated effectiveness against enveloped viruses like herpes simplex and influenza.

Complex and diverse mechanisms, frequently including interactions with components of the virus and the host cell, underlie the antiviral activity of herbal substances. These interactions prevent the virus from replicating, assembling, or entering host cells. Numerous herbal substances target distinct stages of the viral life cycle and inhibit viral infection through complementary routes, hence exhibiting multimodal antiviral activity. Certain herbal compounds have been demonstrated to have direct antiviral effects as well as alter host immunological responses to viral infection. This includes boosting innate antiviral defenses, lowering tissue damage and inflammation linked to viral pathogenesis, and strengthening innate antiviral defenses.

The promise of plant-based medicines as complementary and alternative therapies for the prevention as well as treatment of viral infections is highlighted by the increasing amount of scientific research demonstrating the antiviral qualities of herbal components. To improve the therapeutic efficacy and safety profiles of herbal substances, understand their mechanisms of action, and assess their clinical usefulness in the treatment of viral illnesses, more study is necessary. Plant-based antiviral therapies hold promise for treating viral infections globally and helping to fully realize their therapeutic potential when traditional herbal medicine expertise is combined with cutting-edge scientific approaches.

Herbal Medicine and Modern Healthcare

Previously regarded as supplemental or alternative medicine, herbal therapy is becoming more widely accepted and incorporated into contemporary healthcare systems across the globe. Herbal medicine is the use of plants as well as plant extracts for medicinal purposes; it is also known as botanical medicine or phytotherapy. Clinical practice is guided by scientific research, empirical data, and traditional wisdom. Although the use of herbal remedies has been a part of indigenous healing practices and cultural traditions for thousands of years, there has been a recent surge in interest in herbal medicine that can be attributed to a growing understanding of the potential health benefits of natural remedies as well as a desire for integrative and holistic approaches to healthcare.

Herbal medicine is still widely used in primary healthcare in many parts of the world, especially in areas where access to conventional medical treatments is restricted or prohibitively expensive. For millions of people, traditional healers, herbalists, and community health workers are their main access points to healthcare; they provide herbal cures for a variety of illnesses, from minor ailments to chronic disorders. Families and individuals rely on plants and plant extracts for preventive, supportive, and curative purposes when using herbal medicine in self-care routines and home remedies.

Herbal medicine has become more and more popular not only in traditional and indigenous healing systems but also in mainstream healthcare settings, where it is being incorporated into clinical practice in addition to traditional medical therapies. Herbal medicine is becoming a part of treatment procedures in integrative medicine clinics, wellness centers, and hospitals. This gives patients access to a complete approach to health and healing that integrates the best aspects of complementary and traditional therapies. Increasingly, medical professionals—including doctors, naturopaths, and pharmacists—are obtaining training in herbal medicine and using herbal medicines in their practices, frequently in conjunction with other medical specialists.

The increasing amount of scientific data demonstrating the safety, effectiveness, and therapeutic potential of herbal treatments is one of the leading forces behind the integration of herbal medicine into contemporary healthcare. The identification and characterization of bioactive chemicals in medicinal plants, together with the clarification of their modes of action and pharmacological impacts on human health, have been made possible by advancements in pharmacognosy, phytochemistry, and pharmacology. Important information about the efficacy of herbal medicines for a range of medical illnesses, such as infectious diseases, diabetes, cancer, and cardiovascular disease, has been gleaned via clinical trials, systematic reviews, and meta-analyses.

Compared to traditional medical treatments, herbal therapy has a number of benefits, such as accessibility, affordability, and cultural significance. Due to the widespread availability of herbal medications over-the-counter and online, a diverse variety of people can obtain them, irrespective of their socioeconomic status or geographic location. Generally speaking, herbal remedies are less expensive than pharmaceutical ones, especially in areas with high healthcare expenditures or limited insurance coverage. Moreover, herbal medicine is culturally relevant and acceptable to a wide range of cultures worldwide since it is firmly anchored in indigenous healing practices and cultural traditions.

Herbal medicine faces difficulties in the current healthcare system, such as problems with regulation, standardization, and quality control, despite its increasing acceptability and popularity. The diverse range of herbal products' composition and potency, coupled with the possibility of contamination, adulteration, and mislabeling, emphasizes the necessity of implementing standardized production procedures, quality assurance systems, and regulatory supervision. Concerns regarding adverse effects, contraindications, and herb-drug interactions further emphasize how crucial it is for patients and healthcare professionals to work together to make educated decisions when including herbal treatments in treatment plans.

In summary, there is a resurgence of herbal medicine in contemporary healthcare due to the realization by patients, healthcare professionals, and legislators of the ability of natural medicines to supplement and improve traditional medical therapies. Herbal medicine has the potential to become more and more significant in promoting health, preventing disease, and improving the quality of life for people and communities all over the world by fusing the best aspects of traditional wisdom with contemporary science and evidence-based practice. Herbal medicine will continue to develop and adapt to suit the shifting healthcare demands of a diverse and dynamic global population as research into the therapeutic qualities of medicinal plants advances.

CHAPTER III

Building Your Herbal Toolkit

Identifying and Sourcing Herbs

A vital component of practicing herbal medicine is identifying and procuring plants, which is necessary to guarantee the effectiveness, safety, and quality of herbal medicines. There are several steps in the process, from precisely identifying medicinal plants to ethically obtaining them from reliable vendors or sustainable sources. In order to prevent misidentification and guarantee that the suitable plant species with the intended medicinal characteristics are utilized in herbal remedies, careful identification of herbs is essential. Combining morphological traits like leaf form, flower color, and growth habits with additional diagnostic methods like chemical analysis and genetic testing allows for the accurate identification of plants. Botanical keys, reference books, and internet resources are used by herbalists, botanists, and other qualified specialists to precisely identify medicinal plants and separate them from species that are similar to them or adulterants.

Maintaining the quality and integrity of herbal treatments requires getting herbs from sustainable sources or reputable vendors once they have been accurately identified. When choosing suppliers for the production, collection, and processing of medicinal plants, ethical sourcing techniques emphasize fair trade, sustainability, and environmental care. Because certified organic herbs are grown without the use of artificial pesticides, herbicides, or fertilizers, they are free of dangerous residues and less likely to be contaminated by chemicals when used in herb therapies. Similar to this, wildcrafted herbs are taken from their native environments in a way that respects ecological balance and has the least negative effect possible on populations of wild plants.

In order to guarantee the legitimacy, potency, and purity of herbal products, as well as to avoid adulteration, contamination, or mislabeling, quality control procedures are essential. Tight quality control procedures, including heavy metal screening, microbiological testing, chemical analysis, and botanical identification, should be used by suppliers and producers of herbal treatments. By taking these precautions, herbal products can be guaranteed to meet safety, purity, and efficacy criteria. Additional guarantees of product quality and regulatory compliance are offered by independent third-party testing and certification programs like ConsumerLab.com, NSF International, and the United States Pharmacopeia (USP).

Transparency and accountability are made possible across the supply chain by traceability and documentation, which are crucial components of herbal sourcing. To monitor medicinal plants from field to completed product, suppliers should keep thorough records of botanical origin, growing techniques, harvesting strategies, processing steps, and quality control measures. Herbal goods should be accompanied by certificates of analysis (COAs), batch records, and labeling information that gives consumers vital information on the identity, potency, and purity of the substances.

Medicinal herb cultivation supports regional farmers, communities, and ecosystems while providing a steady supply of high-quality botanicals. Agroforestry methods, permaculture concepts, and organic farming methods can all be used to grow medicinal plants in a way that minimizes adverse environmental effects, preserves biodiversity, and improves soil fertility and health. Small-scale farmers and indigenous groups are enabled to engage in the production and marketing of medicinal herbs through community-based initiatives, cooperative networks, and ethical trading partnerships. This promotes social justice, cultural preservation, and economic growth.

To ensure the long-term sustainability as well as the resilience of natural resources, wildcrafting or the sustainable collection of wild medicinal herbs calls for responsible care of those resources. The ecological integrity of wild plant populations can be preserved while preventing overexploitation and habitat degradation by harvesting rules, seasonal limitations, and conservation measures. Herbalists, wildcrafters, and environmental advocates can contribute to the protection of threatened species, delicate ecosystems, and biodiversity hotspots while guaranteeing a steady supply of wild medicinal herbs for future generations by engaging in responsible wildcrafting and supporting conservation initiatives.

In summary, recognizing and obtaining herbs is a complex process that calls for botanical expertise, moral considerations, and quality control procedures. A thriving herbal medicine industry that supports health, wellness, and environmental stewardship can be fostered by herbalists, suppliers, and consumers by placing a high priority on botanical identification, ethical sourcing, quality control measures, and sustainable cultivation and harvesting techniques. It is imperative that stakeholders—herbalists, botanists, farmers, conservationists, and policymakers—work together to tackle the intricate issues surrounding herbal sourcing and build a more robust and just herbal medicine supply chain.

Basic Principles of Herbal Preparation

Anyone interested in using medicinal plants for health and wellness must grasp the fundamentals of herbal preparation. Herbal preparation refers to a range of techniques used to extract and combine the active ingredients of herbs to make medicinal solutions that can be consumed, administered topically, or breathed. Simple infusions and decoctions to more intricate preparations like tinctures, salves, essential oils, and herbal pills or capsules are among these techniques. Every technique has its own benefits and uses, enabling people to customize their herbal medicines to meet particular health requirements and preferences.

Two of the most popular and straightforward ways to prepare herbs are infusions and decoctions. Herbs are steeped in boiling water to release their soluble components, including vitamins, flavonoids, and essential oils, in an infusion. Infusions are usually employed for sensitive plant components like leaves and flowers. They can be applied topically as compresses, washes, or soaks, or they can be drunk as herbal teas. Conversely, in order to extract therapeutic compounds from more challenging plant parts like seeds, bark, and roots, they must be simmered in water for a more extended period of time. Decoctions are frequently employed to prepare herbal remedies with more potent therapeutic effects since they are better suited for extracting water-insoluble components.

Another well-liked technique for preparing herbal remedies is tincturing, which entails utilizing alcohol or a combination of alcohol and water to extract the therapeutic properties of herbs. In contrast to infusions or decoctions, tinctures are highly concentrated liquid extracts that maintain the active ingredients of plants and have a longer shelf life. They are convenient and simple to administer because they can be taken orally by diluting them in water or other beverages. Additionally, tinctures can be topically administered to the skin to provide localized relief from skin problems, inflammation, or pain. The alcohol in tinctures acts as a preservative and makes it easier to extract the components from the plants that are soluble in alcohol as well as water.

Herbs can be used to generate semi-solid or solid formulations, such as herbal oils and salves, by infusing them in carrier oils or mixing them with additional components like beeswax. Salves are applied directly to relieve and heal skin irritations, wounds, or bug bites, while herbal oils are frequently used for massage, aromatherapy, or as the foundation for skincare products. The process of making herbal oils involves macerating herbs in carrier oils, including olive, coconut, or almond oil, and then allowing the infusion to steep for some time before straining out the plant material. Heat infusion techniques can also be used to make herbal oils to expedite the extraction process.

Essential oils are concentrated aromatic chemicals obtained from plants via solvent extraction, steam distillation, or cold pressing. Essential oils are highly valued for their medicinal qualities and are applied topically in aromatherapy, massage, and inhalation. Every essential oil has distinct qualities and advantages, varying from sedative and antibacterial to analgesic and anti-inflammatory. Essential oils may be used as they are or in combination with other essential oils, plant extracts, or carrier oils to create customized mixtures for certain emotional or health needs. When utilizing essential oils, care must be taken because they are strong and, if not handled correctly, might result in skin irritation or other adverse effects.

For those who would rather take their herbal supplements in a more standardized and portable form, herbal capsules and tablets offer a convenient dose form. Herbs are dried and ground into fine powders for these formulations, which are then compressed or enclosed in tablets. For herbs that are bitter or unpleasant, such as teas or tinctures, herbal capsules, and tablets are usually utilized, as they facilitate easy administration and accurate dosage. However, to guarantee potency, purity, and safety, it's crucial to select premium supplements from reliable producers.

In conclusion, people can harness the healing potential of plants for their health and well-being by knowing the fundamentals of herbal preparation. To get the best results when creating herbal teas, tinctures, oils, salves, essential oils, or capsules, it's vital to choose high-quality herbs, follow dosage recommendations, and employ the proper extraction techniques. People can naturally promote holistic well-being, address specific health conditions, and improve their general health by adding herbal remedies to their healthcare regimens. To guarantee the safe and efficient use of medicinal herbs, it is imperative that you see a trained herbalist or healthcare professional before starting any herbal treatment, particularly if you have any underlying medical issues or are on medication.

Herbal Formulations and Combinations

Comprehending the blends and arrangements of herbs is crucial to optimizing the therapeutic advantages of medicinal plants and crafting efficacious herbal treatments. The precise mixtures of herbs and other substances used to make herbal treatments, such as teas, tinctures, oils, salves, capsules, and tablets, are referred to as herbal formulations. These combinations can differ significantly based on the intended therapeutic benefits, the characteristics of the herbs employed, and the preferences of the herbalist or healthcare professional. They are frequently based on traditional knowledge, empirical data, and scientific study.

A single herb is used to treat a particular health issue or symptom in a single-herb preparation, which is one of the most popular kinds of herbal formulations. The selection of single-herb formulations is frequently guided by the herb's known pharmacological characteristics, historical use, and verifiable efficacy. Single-herb formulations include echinacea tincture for immune support, arnica salve for pain relief and bruising, and chamomile tea for relaxation and sleep support. When addressing a particular health concern or for people who are intolerant to certain herbs, single-herb mixtures can be beneficial.

However, in order to maximize their therapeutic effects and treat several facets of health and wellness at once, many herbal therapies combine several plants. A variety of elements, such as contemporary pharmacological research, clinical experience, and traditional herbal medicine systems, can be used to construct herbal combinations. In order to provide a more thorough and well-rounded therapeutic strategy, herbalists frequently blend plants with complementary activities or synergistic effects. Herbs that have adaptogenic qualities, such as holy basil, Rhodiola, and ashwagandha, are frequently mixed to assist the body's reaction to stress and to encourage general resilience and vigor.

Herbal combinations are frequently given in traditional herbal medicine systems, such as Ayurveda, Traditional Chinese Medicine (TCM), and Western herbalism, based on constitutional types, pattern distinctions, and customized treatment protocols. Herbal remedies are designed explicitly in Ayurveda to balance the three doshas (Pitta, Kapha, and Vata) to treat particular imbalances or illnesses. To help the body regain balance and harmony, traditional Chinese medicine (TCM) formulates herbal combinations using the yin and yang, five elements, and the meridian system as guiding principles. Herbal combinations in Western herbalism can be created depending on the individual's symptoms and constitution, as well as the particular activities and energetics of the plants.

Additionally, herbal concoctions can be made to target organ systems or bodily physiological processes specifically. Herbs that have hepatic and cholagogic qualities, such as artichoke leaf, dandelion root, and milk thistle, are frequently mixed to support the health of the liver and gallbladder as well as to aid in detoxification and digestion. Similarly, kidney and urinary tract function can be supported, and sensations of pain or inflammation in the urine can be reduced by combining herbs that have diuretic and antispasmodic qualities, such as marshmallow root, cleavers, and parsley.

Herbal synergy combinations can reduce the possibility of adverse responses or side effects while maximizing the medicinal benefits of individual herbs. Certain herbs have the ability to act as potentiators, meaning they can improve the activity, bioavailability, or absorption of other herbs in the mixture. In herbal formulations, for instance, black pepper extract (piperine) is frequently used to boost the bioavailability of curcumin from turmeric, hence augmenting its anti-inflammatory and antioxidant properties. To provide a more harmonic and balanced therapeutic result, additional herbs may function as modulators, adjusting or balancing the effects of other herbs.

Combining herbs can be dangerous, though, as some combinations might worsen preexisting medical issues or interfere with medicine. When creating herbal treatments for patients or customers, herbalists and medical professionals should take into account any potential drug interactions, contraindications, and individual sensitivities. When utilizing herbal mixtures, it's also crucial to start with moderate doses and keep an eye out for any unexpected effects or bad reactions, especially in sensitive groups like youngsters, the elderly, and those who are pregnant or nursing.

In conclusion, developing safe and effective herbal medicines that address the intricate and multidimensional aspects of health and wellness requires a grasp of herbal formulations and combinations. Choosing premium herbs, following the proper preparation methods, and customizing the medicine to the patient's requirements and preferences are crucial when employing either single- herb preparations or herbal combos. Herbalists and healthcare professionals can maximize the therapeutic benefits of medicinal plants and advance holistic health and well-being by combining the synergistic effects of several herbs in well-considered and evidence-based formulations. To improve our understanding of herbal combinations and formulations and incorporate them into standard medical practice, traditional herbalists, contemporary researchers, and healthcare professionals must work together.

Safety Guidelines and Precautions

It is essential to take safety precautions and standards into account when utilizing herbal treatments to support well-being and health. Although there are many advantages to using herbal medicine, such as natural healing, symptom relief, and general well-being, it is crucial to use caution and be aware of any potential hazards and contraindications. Safety instructions cover a wide range of topics, such as choosing high-quality herbs, administering them correctly and at the correct dosage, being aware of any possible interactions or side effects, and seeking the advice of licensed healthcare providers when necessary.

Choosing premium herbs from reliable suppliers is one of the cornerstones of herbal safety. High-quality herbs are devoid of pesticides, heavy metals, and other pollutants and are produced, harvested, and processed using ethical and sustainable methods. Herbal medicines can be consumed safely and effectively if they meet quality and purity standards, which can be achieved by organic certification or independent testing. Furthermore, in order to avoid misidentification or adulteration, it is crucial to confirm the identity and authenticity of herbs using botanical identification and quality control procedures.

The correct use and administration of herbal remedies are crucial for their safety since misuse or overdosing can result in harmful effects or toxicity. Recommendations for dosage are frequently given by herbalists, medical professionals, and manufacturers, drawing from scientific study, clinical experience, and traditional usage. It's critical to carefully read these instructions and begin with small doses, particularly if you're trying a new herb or combination of herbs. When establishing the dosage and frequency of administration, individual parameters such as age, weight, medical history, and herb sensitivity should also be taken into account.

It's crucial to comprehend possible interactions and adverse effects in order to reduce dangers and guarantee the secure use of herbal medicines. Although herbs are typically regarded as safe when used as directed, some people may experience adverse side effects, mainly when using high doses or for prolonged periods of time. Herbal treatments frequently cause allergic responses, upset stomachs, headaches, dizziness, and skin irritation as adverse effects. Furthermore, there is a chance that herbs will interfere with prescription drugs, dietary supplements, or underlying medical issues, which could have negative consequences. Prior to using herbs, it's essential to learn about any possible interactions or side effects and to speak with a licensed healthcare provider if you have any questions or concerns.

When utilizing herbal treatments, specific populations—such as those who are pregnant or nursing, toddlers, elderly adults, and people with pre-existing medical conditions—may need to take extra precautions. Herbal remedies should be used with caution by those who are pregnant or nursing, as some of them may have hormonal or uterine-stimulating effects that could harm the unborn child or the mother. Because of their more diminutive stature and still-developing physiology, children may be more vulnerable to the effects of herbs; therefore, it's crucial to use lower doses and see a pediatrician before giving children any herbs. An older adult's body may react differently to herbal medicines because of diminished metabolic capacity or weakened organ function. Before utilizing herbal medicines, people with pre-existing medical illnesses such as diabetes, autoimmune diseases, liver or renal disease, or kidney disease should also speak with a healthcare provider because some herbs can interact with pharmaceuticals or make underlying medical conditions worse.

The use of herbal treatments is subject to generic safety measures in addition to particular concerns. Storing herbs properly in a cool, dry place away from sunshine and moisture is one way to preserve their effectiveness and freshness. The administration and preparation instructions, which include dosage calculations, brewing durations, and suitable dilution, must also be carefully followed. Keep children and pets away from herbal treatments to avoid misuse or unintentional intake. Herbal therapies should never be used if you encounter any adverse side effects or unexpected results. If needed, get medical help right away.

To sum up, safety protocols and safeguards are critical to guaranteeing the secure and efficient application of herbal treatments to enhance health and well-being. People can reduce risks and enhance the advantages of herbal medicine by choosing high-quality herbs, adhering to specified dosage guidelines, being aware of potential side effects and interactions, and seeking the advice of experienced healthcare professionals when necessary.

Although using herbs can be a natural and holistic therapeutic alternative, it is essential to employ caution, awareness, and respect for the potential consequences on the body when using them. Herbal medicines have the potential to be effective instruments for promoting general health and well-being when used correctly and with safety precautions taken.

CHAPTER IV

Herbal Solutions for Specific Viral Infections

Influenza and Common Cold

Since ancient times, people have utilized herbal remedies to treat the common cold and influenza in order to reduce symptoms, strengthen the immune system, and encourage the body's inherent healing mechanisms. Both the common cold and influenza sometimes referred to as the flu, are viral respiratory infections, albeit they differ in terms of intensity, duration, and specific symptoms. Herbal medicine provides a comprehensive strategy that treats the underlying causes of sickness and enhances general well-being, in contrast to traditional treatments for similar conditions, which usually concentrate on symptom management and antiviral drugs. A variety of herbs, botanical extracts, and traditional formulations are used in herbal remedies for influenza and the common cold to address symptoms like fever, congestion, coughing, sore throats, and fatigue. These remedies also support immune system function, reduce inflammation, and improve respiratory health.

Echinacea is among the most well-known plants used to treat colds and the flu. Echinacea is highly valued for strengthening the immune system and reducing the length and intensity of respiratory illnesses. According to studies, echinacea extracts can boost the body's defenses against viral infections, boost the immune system, and improve the generation of white blood cells. When colds and flu first appear, echinacea can be given as a tincture, capsule, tea, or lozenge to help prevent sickness or decrease its duration.

Elderberry is another famous herb used to treat respiratory infections. For ages, elderberries have been used in traditional medicine to treat fever, coughing, and congestion associated with colds and the flu. Potent antioxidants, flavonoids, and anthocyanins found in elderberry extracts have antiviral qualities and support a healthy immune system. Taking an elderberry supplement can lessen the length and intensity of cold and flu symptoms, as well as assist in shielding the body against viral infections. Convenient and efficient ways to use elderberry in a cold and flu treatment routine are syrup, lozenges, and capsules.

Another adaptable herb that's frequently used to treat respiratory infections, the flu, and colds is ginger. The natural anti-inflammatory, antiviral, and expectorant qualities of ginger help reduce symptoms like fever, sore throat, congestion, and cough. Ginger tea, prepared by brewing fresh ginger slices in a pot of hot water, provides a comforting and soothing remedy that can help improve respiratory symptoms and overall well-being when taken during an illness. Soups, stews, and other meals can benefit from the flavor-enhancing and additional therapeutic properties of ginger added to them.

Garlic is another powerful plant that works wonders for colds and the flu because of its antiviral, antibacterial, and immune-boosting qualities. Garlic carries a substance called allicin, which has been shown to inhibit the growth of germs and viruses and strengthen the immune system's response against disease. When cold or flu symptoms first appear, eating raw garlic or taking supplements containing garlic may help lessen the intensity and duration of the sickness as well as assist in avoiding getting sick again. For ease, garlic can be taken as a supplement or added to soups, salads, and other meals.

Another herb that is frequently used in traditional medicine to treat respiratory infections, the flu, and colds is licorice root. Licorice root relieves cough, sore throat, and congestion because it includes chemicals with antiviral, expectorant, and anti-inflammatory qualities. Extracting the medicinal components of licorice root can be prepared as a decoction or brewed from dried slices of licorice root. Supplements containing licorice root are now offered in capsule or tincture form for individuals who want a more convenient and concentrated solution.

Peppermint, eucalyptus, thyme, and oregano are other herbs that are frequently used in herbal therapies for colds and flu. These herbs contain antibacterial, expectorant, and immune-boosting qualities that help reduce respiratory symptoms and promote general health. For the purpose of clearing congestion and making breathing easier, eucalyptus essential oil can be used topically or used in steam inhalations. Peppermint tea is a calming remedy for sore throats and congestion. Strong antibacterial properties found in thyme and oregano aid in the prevention of infections and strengthen the immune system, making them beneficial complements to herbal remedies for the common cold and flu.

Herbal mixtures and formulations are frequently utilized in addition to single herbs to increase the potency of herbal treatments for the flu and colds. Combining different herbs with complementary activities allows herbalists and healthcare professionals to address a broader range of symptoms and offer more thorough support for respiratory and immune system health. Herbs that enhance general health and vitality, as well as those that have antiviral, immune-boosting, expectorant, and anti-inflammatory qualities, can be found in herbal formulations. Herbal teas, tinctures, syrups, and capsules that combine immune-boosting herbs like echinacea, elderberry, and astragalus with expectorant and calming herbs like ginger, licorice, and thyme are a few examples of herbal combinations for colds and flu.

Herbal medicines can be helpful in treating the flu and colds, but for best results, take them sparingly and in conjunction with other supporting measures. The body needs help from its immune system, and recovering from illness can be made easier by eating a nutritious diet, reducing stress, getting adequate sleep, and drinking plenty of water. It's also essential to see a qualified healthcare professional before starting any herbal therapy, especially if you have any underlying medical conditions or are on medication, to ensure the safe and effective use of medicinal herbs. Herbal remedies for the flu and colds can be valuable instruments for promoting general health and well-being if used correctly and with caution.

Herpes Viruses

A class of DNA viruses known as herpes viruses is responsible for a number of illnesses in humans, such as shingles, chickenpox, vaginal and oral herpes, and Epstein-Barr virus (EBV). These viruses are highly contagious and can also be spread by direct contact with those who have them, as well as by contact with contaminated objects or human fluids. Herbal therapy provides a variety of natural treatments that can help control symptoms, lessen the frequency and intensity of outbreaks, and enhance immune system performance, even though there is presently no known cure for herpes viruses.

One of the plants that have been studied the most for treating herpes viruses is lemon balm (Melissa officinalis). Flavonoids and rosmarinic acid, two antiviral chemicals found in lemon balm, have been demonstrated to impede the herpes simplex viruses (HSV-1) reproduction and lessen the frequency and length of outbreaks of genital herpes and cold sores (HSV-1). While dietary supplementation with lemon balm extract or tea may help avoid outbreaks and promote faster healing, topical application of lemon balm ointment or cream can help soothe and treat sores.

Echinacea (Echinacea purpurea) is another herb that is frequently used in herbal therapies for herpes viruses. Echinacea is highly valued for its capacity to strengthen the body's defenses against viral infections and to increase immunity. According to studies, echinacea extracts help lessen the intensity and length of colds, the flu, and other viral diseases, as well as boost the formation of white blood cells and immune cell activity. Echinacea can be consumed orally as a tea, tincture, or tablet to boost immunity and stop herpes outbreaks.

Another herb with antiviral qualities that is frequently included in herbal treatments for herpes viruses is licorice root (Glycyrrhiza glabra). Glycyrrhizin, a substance found in licorice root, has been demonstrated to impede the reproduction of HSV and other viruses by preventing viral attachment to and entry into host cells. Oral licorice root extract supplementation may help prevent outbreaks and minimize viral shedding. In contrast, topical application of licorice root ointment or cream might help relieve discomfort, inflammation, and itching associated with herpes blisters.

Another herb with antiviral solid qualities that can aid in the fight against herpes viruses is olive leaf (Olea europaea). Oleuropein, a substance found in olive leaves, has been demonstrated to impede the reproduction of HSV and other viruses by interfering with the mechanisms involved in viral assembly and replication. According to studies, olive leaf extract may be able to lessen the frequency and intensity of herpes outbreaks as well as stop the virus from spreading to other people. As a tea, tincture, or pill, olive leaf extract can be consumed orally to boost immunity and lower viral activity.

Since ancient times, propolis, a resinous material made by honeybees, has been utilized in traditional medicine for its immune-stimulating and antibacterial qualities. Flavonoids, phenolic acids, and other bioactive substances found in propolis have been demonstrated to suppress the growth of HSV and other viruses while enhancing the function of immune cells. Oral propolis extract or tincture intake may help prevent outbreaks and enhance immunological function, while topical application of propolis ointment or cream can help soothe and treat herpes sores.

Due to its immune-boosting and antiviral qualities, astragalus root (Astragalus membranaceus) is a herb that is frequently used in traditional Chinese medicine (TCM). Polysaccharides, flavonoids, and saponins found in astragalus have been demonstrated to improve immunological response, boost leukemic cell formation, and impede virus replication. Astragalus root supports immune function and lessens the frequency and intensity of herpes outbreaks when taken orally as a tea, tincture, or capsule.

Another traditional Chinese herb that has been utilized for generations due to its immune-modulating and antiviral effects is reishi mushroom (Ganoderma lucidum). Polysaccharides, triterpenes, and other bioactive substances found in reishi have been demonstrated to improve immunological response, lessen inflammatory response, and impede the growth of viruses. Research has indicated that reishi mushroom extract may be able to lessen the frequency and intensity of herpes outbreaks as well as perhaps stop the virus from spreading to other people. Reishi mushroom extract can be consumed orally as a tea, tincture, or tablet to boost defenses against viruses.

Herbal combinations and formulations are frequently utilized in addition to single herbs to increase the efficacy of herbal treatments for herpes viruses. Herbalists and medical professionals can blend several herbs with complementary properties to treat a wider variety of symptoms, strengthen the immune system, and offer more thorough support to people with herpes infections. Herbal remedies for herpes viruses can take the form of topical ointments or creams that contain a mixture of extracts from lemon balm, licorice root, and propolis to heal and soothe lesions, or they can be taken as oral supplements that contain extracts from echinacea, olive leaf, astragalus, and reishi mushrooms to boost immunity and lower viral activity.

Herbal therapies have the potential to manage herpes viruses effectively; nevertheless, for best outcomes, they should be used responsibly and in conjunction with other supporting measures. The body's immune system has to be supported, as well as general health and well-being, by appropriate nutrition, stress reduction, adequate sleep, and decent hygiene. It's also essential to see a qualified healthcare professional before starting any herbal therapy, especially if you have any underlying medical conditions or are on medication, to ensure the safe and effective use of medicinal herbs. Herbal remedies for herpes viruses can be valuable tools for treating symptoms, preventing outbreaks, and enhancing general health and wellness when used correctly and with caution.

Respiratory Syncytial Virus (RSV)

Common respiratory viruses like the respiratory syncytial virus (RSV) can cause mild to severe respiratory illnesses, particularly in young children, older people, and people with compromised immune systems. RSV infections usually cause cold-like symptoms, such as fever, runny nose, coughing, and difficulty breathing; however, in more severe cases—particularly in newborns and early children—they can cause pneumonia and bronchiolitis. Herbal therapy offers a variety of natural therapies that can help reduce symptoms, strengthen immune function, and improve respiratory health, even if there isn't a specific antiviral drug available for RSV at this time.

One of the most popular herbs for treating respiratory infections, including RSV, is elderberry (Sambucus nigra). Elderberry has long been used in traditional medicine to boost immunity and lessen the symptoms of respiratory illnesses like the flu and colds. Potent antioxidants and flavonoids found in elderberry extracts have been demonstrated to stop the spread of viruses, including RSV, and to lessen respiratory tract inflammation. Supplementing with elderberries has been shown in studies to reduce the length and intensity of respiratory infections as well as their potential to prevent complications like pneumonia.

Another well-liked plant used in herbal treatments for respiratory infections, such as RSV, is echinacea (Echinacea purpurea). White blood cell production is stimulated by echinacea's immune-boosting qualities, which also strengthen the body's defenses against viral infections. Research has demonstrated that by enhancing immune function and decreasing inflammation, echinacea extracts can lessen the intensity and length of colds, the flu, and other respiratory diseases. Echinacea can be consumed orally as a tea, tincture, or tablet to boost immunity and lower the risk of complications from RSV infection.

Another herb that's frequently used in herbal therapies for respiratory infections like RSV is licorice root (Glycyrrhiza glabra). Compounds included in licorice root have antiviral and anti-inflammatory qualities that aid in respiratory tract healing and calm the respiratory system while lowering inflammation and coughing. It has been shown that the compound glycyrrhizin, found in licorice root, suppresses the growth of respiratory viruses, including RSV, by keeping the virus from adhering to and infiltrating host cells. To relieve the symptoms of an RSV infection, licorice root can be applied locally as a gargle or throat spray or consumed orally as a tincture, pill, or tea.

The adaptable plant ginger (Zingiber officinale) is frequently employed in herbal treatments for respiratory infections because of its expectorant, antibacterial, and anti-inflammatory qualities. Ginger includes substances called gingerol and shogaol that facilitate easier breathing, lessen coughing and congestion, and reduce respiratory tract irritation. In addition to promoting general respiratory health, ginger tea, which is prepared by steeping fresh ginger slices in hot water, is a calming and warming therapy that can help ease RSV infection symptoms.

Due to its antibacterial and expectorant properties, thyme (Thymus vulgaris) is a fragrant herb that is effective in treating respiratory infections, including RSV. Thyme includes volatile oils, like carvacrol and thymol, which have been demonstrated to help break up mucus in the respiratory tract and prevent the formation of bacteria and viruses. Thyme tea, prepared by steeping dried thyme leaves in hot water, has several benefits, including relieving sore throats, easing congestion and coughing, and improving respiratory health. In order to reduce the symptoms of an RSV infection, thyme essential oil can also be applied topically or through steam inhalations.

Another plant with antibacterial solid qualities that can help fight RSV and other respiratory viruses is oregano (Origanum vulgare). Carvacrol and thymol, two substances found in oregano, have been demonstrated to suppress the growth of germs and viruses and strengthen the immune system. Oregano tea, made by steeping dried oregano leaves in hot water, can help ease symptoms of an RSV infection, including cough, congestion, and sore throat. To support respiratory health and lessen the symptoms of respiratory infections, oregano essential oil can also be used topically or applied via steam inhalation or chest massages.

Herbal formulations and combinations are frequently utilized in addition to single herbs to increase the efficacy of herbal treatments for RSV and other respiratory diseases. Herbalists and medical professionals can blend several herbs that have complementary properties to address a wider variety of symptoms, strengthen the immune system, and offer more all-encompassing support for respiratory health. Herbal teas, tinctures, syrups, and capsules containing a combination of elderberry, echinacea, licorice root, ginger, thyme, and oregano extracts to relieve symptoms, lower inflammation, and boost immunity are a few examples of herbal combinations for RSV.

Herbal medicines have the potential to manage RSV symptoms and improve respiratory health effectively, but for best outcomes, they should be used responsibly and in conjunction with other supportive measures. To boost the immune system and expedite the healing process from respiratory infections, it is imperative to adhere to proper hygiene habits, adequate rest, hydration, and nutrition. It's also essential to see a qualified healthcare professional before starting any herbal therapy, especially if you have any underlying medical conditions or are on medication, to ensure the safe and effective use of medicinal herbs. Herbal remedies for RSV can be valuable tools for symptom relief, immune system support, and the promotion of general respiratory health and well-being when used correctly and with caution.

Human Immunodeficiency Virus (HIV)

Herbal remedies for the Human Immunodeficiency Virus (HIV) have attracted a lot of attention as alternatives to and complements to traditional antiretroviral therapy (ART). HIV is a retrovirus that targets particular CD4 T cells to eliminate immunological cells. This results in immunodeficiency and heightened vulnerability to opportunistic infections and cancers. Though stopping viral replication and increasing life expectancy, antiretroviral therapy (ART) has transformed the way HIV/AIDS is managed. However, ART is not without side effects, medication resistance, and difficulties maintaining long-term adherence. Herbal medicine provides a wide range of natural medicines that may boost immune system performance, reduce symptoms, and enhance general health in HIV-positive persons.

Astragalus (Astragalus membranaceus) is one of the herbs concerning HIV/AIDS that has been researched the most. A traditional Chinese herb, astragalus is prized for its adaptogenic and immune-boosting qualities. According to studies, astragalus extracts include polysaccharides and saponins that can boost CD4 T cell numbers, improve immunological function, and stop HIV-infected cells from replicating the virus. Furthermore, astragalus may help lessen oxidative stress, inflammation, and HIV-related symptoms like lethargy, diarrhea, and weight loss. Although further research is required to determine its safety and efficacy, astragalus is frequently used in herbal formulations for the support of HIV/AIDS.

Another plant that may be beneficial to people living with HIV/AIDS is a cat's Claw (Uncaria tomentosa). Indigenous societies have long utilized the woody vine known as "cat's claw," which is native to the Amazon rainforest, for its antiviral, immunomodulatory, and anti-inflammatory qualities. Alkaloids, glycosides, and other bioactive substances found In cat's claws have been demonstrated to ease HIV/AIDS symptoms, lower viral loads, and strengthen immune systems. Cat's Claw may also improve general health and well-being and lessen the adverse effects of antiretroviral therapy (ART), such as gastrointestinal distress and immunological reconstitution syndrome (IRIS).

Another plant that has been researched for its possible advantages in managing HIV/AIDS is garlic (Allium sativum). Allicin, a sulfur-based molecule with antioxidant, immunomodulatory, and antibacterial qualities, is found in garlic. Garlic supplementation has been linked in studies to improved immune function, decreased viral loads, and increased CD4 T cell counts in HIV/AIDS patients. Garlic may also help reduce the symptoms of opportunistic infections, heart problems, and metabolic issues related to HIV/AIDS and antiretroviral therapy. Garlic is frequently used in food and medicine due to its possible health advantages, although further research is required to validate its efficacy and safety.

The popular herb echinacea, also known as echinacea purpurea, is well-known for strengthening the immune system and promoting the body's defenses against viral infections. Polysaccharides, flavonoids, and alkamides found in echinacea have been demonstrated to improve white blood cell formation, boost immunity, and lessen the intensity and duration of viral diseases such as the flu and colds. Although there hasn't been much research on echinacea, especially in relation to HIV/AIDS, it might be helpful for boosting immune system performance and lowering viral replication in those who are HIV/AIDS positive. Herbal compositions for immune support and overall well-being frequently contain echinacea.

Another herb that has been studied for possible benefits in HIV/AIDS management is licorice root (Glycyrrhiza glabra). Glycyrrhizin, a substance found in licorice root, has antiviral, anti-inflammatory, and immunomodulatory qualities. Research has indicated that extracts from licorice roots may help prevent HIV replication, lessen oxidative stress and inflammation, and enhance immunological response in HIV/AIDS patients. Furthermore, licorice root may help reduce HIV/AIDS and ART-related symptoms like fatigue, diarrhea, and oral thrush. Although further studies are required to verify its safety and effectiveness, licorice root is frequently included in herbal formulations for HIV/AIDS support.

The spice and medicinal herb turmeric (Curcuma longa) is well-known for its anti-inflammatory, antioxidant, and also immunomodulatory qualities. Curcumin, a bioactive substance found in turmeric, has been demonstrated to lessen inflammation, stop the spread of viruses, and enhance immune system performance in HIV/AIDS patients. Research has indicated that curcumin administration could potentially lower viral loads, boost CD4 T cell counts, and alleviate symptoms in HIV/AIDS patients. Turmeric may also lessen ART side effects, including gastrointestinal distress, liver damage, and inflammation. Because of its possible health advantages, turmeric is frequently employed in culinary and pharmaceutical preparations, while further research is required to confirm its usefulness and safety.

Herbal formulations and combinations are frequently utilized in addition to single herbs to increase the efficacy of herbal treatments for HIV/AIDS. Herbalists and medical professionals can blend several herbs with complementary properties to treat a wider variety of symptoms, strengthen the immune system, and offer more all-encompassing care to HIV/AIDS patients. Herbal teas, tinctures, capsules, and powders containing a combination of immune-boosting herbs like Astragalus, Cat's Claw, Garlic, Echinacea, Licorice root, and Turmeric are a few examples of herbal combinations for HIV/AIDS. These herbal remedies may assist those living with

HIV/AIDS in enhancing their immune system, lowering their viral load, managing their symptoms, and generally living better.

While using herbal medicines in conjunction with traditional medical care might be beneficial for those living with HIV/AIDS, it's crucial to use them properly. Herbal medicine should be used as a supplemental strategy to enhance immune function, reduce symptoms, and enhance general well-being, not as an alternative to antiretroviral therapy (ART) or other recommended therapies for HIV/AIDS. To guarantee the safe and efficient use of medicinal herbs, you should also speak with a skilled healthcare provider before beginning any herbal remedy, particularly if you have any underlying medical conditions or are on medication. Herbal remedies for HIV/AIDS can be valuable tools for boosting immune function, lowering viral load, and improving general health and well-being in those living with the disease if they are used correctly and with regard to safety concerns.

Hepatitis Viruses

One family of viruses that primarily affects the liver is known as the hepatitis virus, which damages and inflames liver cells. Hepatitis A, B, C, D, and also E are among the various varieties of hepatitis viruses; each has a unique route of transmission, severity, and course of treatment. While supportive care and antiviral drugs are standard components of conventional therapies for hepatitis viruses, herbal therapy provides a variety of natural remedies that can support liver function, lessen inflammation, and enhance general health in hepatitis patients.

Milk thistle (Silybum marianum), one of the most well-known herbs for liver health, is often used in herbal remedies for hepatitis viruses. A substance found in milk thistle called silymarin has anti-inflammatory and antioxidant qualities that help shield liver cells from harm and encourage regeneration. Research has demonstrated that taking supplements containing milk thistle can help people with hepatitis B and C feel better, reduce inflammation in their livers, and improve liver function tests. Furthermore, milk thistle may help avoid liver damage brought on by drugs, alcohol, and pollutants.

Because of its liver-protective and detoxifying qualities, dandelion root (Taraxacum officinale) is another herb that is frequently used in herbal treatments for hepatitis viruses. Sesquiterpene lactones, which are bitter substances found in dandelion roots, increase bile flow and production, enhancing liver and digestive functions.

Furthermore, the antioxidants and vitamins included in dandelion root help shield liver cells from the harm that oxidative stress and inflammation may do. Supplementing with dandelion root has been demonstrated in studies to help lower liver enzyme levels, enhance liver function, and lessen symptoms in those suffering from hepatitis B and C.

Traditional Chinese herb Schisandra (Schisandra chinensis) is prized for its hepatoprotective and adaptogenic qualities. Lignans and other bioactive substances found in Schisandra aid in controlling liver function, lowering inflammation, and shielding liver cells from harm. Supplementing with Schisandra has been found in studies to help lower liver inflammation, enhance liver function tests, and lessen symptoms in those suffering from hepatitis B and C. Furthermore, Schisandra may improve overall well-being and immunological function in those with chronic liver disease.

Because of its liver-supporting and cleansing qualities, burdock root (Arctium lappa) is a frequent therapeutic herb in traditional herbal medicine applications. Inulin and mucilage, two bitter substances found in burdock root, help to stimulate the production and flow of bile, which facilitates the removal of waste and toxins from the liver and gallbladder. Burdock root also contains a wealth of vitamins and antioxidants that help shield liver cells from oxidative stress and inflammation. According to studies, taking supplements containing burdock root can help people with hepatitis B and also C feel better, reduce inflammation in their livers, and improve liver function tests.

Because of its antiviral and anti-inflammatory qualities, licorice root (Glycyrrhiza glabra) is another herb that is frequently used in herbal therapies for hepatitis viruses. Glycyrrhizin, a substance found in licorice root, has been demonstrated to lessen liver inflammation and stop the hepatitis B and C viruses from replicating. Furthermore, the antioxidants and flavonoids included in licorice root help shield liver cells from the harm that oxidative stress and inflammation may do. Research has demonstrated that supplementing with licorice root can help patients with hepatitis B and C feel better, reduce inflammation in the liver, and improve liver function tests.

The spice and medicinal herb turmeric (Curcuma longa) is well-known for its hepatoprotective, antioxidant, and anti-inflammatory qualities. Curcumin, a bioactive substance found in turmeric, has been demonstrated to lessen hepatitis B and C viral multiplication, lessen hepatitis C inflammation, and shield liver cells from oxidative stress and inflammation-related damage. Research has demonstrated that taking a turmeric supplement can help people with hepatitis B and also Hepatitis C feel better, reduce inflammation in the liver, and improve liver function tests. Turmeric may also improve overall health and immune system performance in people with chronic liver disease.

Herbal formulations and combinations are frequently utilized in addition to single herbs to increase the efficacy of herbal treatments for hepatitis viruses. Herbalists and medical professionals may blend different herbs with complementary properties to treat a wider variety of hepatitis symptoms, enhance liver function, and enhance general health. Herbal teas, tinctures, pills, and powders containing a combination of liver-supporting herbs such as milk thistle, dandelion root, schisandra, burdock root, licorice root, and turmeric are a few examples of herbal combinations for hepatitis viruses. These herbal remedies may lessen inflammation, enhance liver function, shield liver cells from harm, and ease hepatitis virus-related symptoms.

Although using herbal medicines in conjunction with traditional medical care can be beneficial for those with hepatitis viruses, it's crucial to utilize them properly. Herbal medicine can be used to maintain liver function, reduce inflammation, and enhance general well-being. Still, it shouldn't be used in place of antiviral drugs or other prescribed therapies for hepatitis viruses. To guarantee the safe and efficient use of medicinal herbs, you should also speak with a skilled healthcare provider before beginning any herbal remedy, particularly if you have any underlying medical conditions or are on medication. Herbal remedies for hepatitis viruses can be proper instruments for promoting liver health and enhancing the quality of life in people with hepatitis, provided they are correctly used, and safety precautions are taken.

Emerging Viral Threats (e.g., Zika, Ebola)

Herbal remedies for newly developing viral dangers, like Ebola and Zika, offer a viable way to supplement traditional medical treatments and deal with the problems these infectious diseases present. While immunizations and antiviral medications remain essential components of containment strategies for outbreaks, herbal therapy offers a plethora of natural remedies that can strengthen immune system function, lessen symptoms, and enhance overall health in patients afflicted with these viruses.

The Zika virus, first identified in 1947 in Uganda, gained global recognition in 2015–2016 as a result of an outbreak in the Americas. Though it can also spread from mother to fetus through blood transfusions, pregnancy, and sexual activity, the primary way that Zika is spread occurs via the sting caused by an infected Aedes mosquito. Severe birth problems, including microcephaly, can result from Zika. Although there isn't a specific antiviral drug available for Zika at this time, herbal medicines can help with immune system support and symptom management. Herbs, including licorice root, echinacea, elderberry, and garlic, that have antiviral and immune-boosting qualities, may help lessen inflammation, hasten healing, and lessen the intensity and duration of Zika symptoms.

Comparably, Ebola virus disease (EVD) was first discovered in 1976 following outbreaks in Sudan and the Democratic Republic of the Congo. It is a severe and frequently fatal illness brought on by the Ebola virus. The Ebola virus can be transmitted by direct contact with the blood, body fluids, or tissues of an infected person or animal. This can lead to a severe hemorrhagic fever with a high fatality rate. Even though there are experimental cures and vaccinations for Ebola, in countries with limited resources, access to these interventions may be restricted during epidemics. Herbal treatments such as olive leaf extract, Astragalus, ginger, and turmeric have antiviral, immuno-boosting, and anti-inflammatory qualities that may help strengthen immune function, lessen viral replication, and relieve symptoms in Ebola virus disease patients.

Due to its many uses in herbal medicine, ginger (Zingiber officinale) is a multipurpose herb with anti-inflammatory, antibacterial, and immune-boosting qualities. Bioactive substances found in ginger, such as shogaol and gingerol, have been demonstrated to enhance immune system performance, lessen inflammation, and prevent the spread of viruses. Research has indicated that taking supplements containing ginger may help lessen the intensity and length of viral infections, as well as their associated symptoms, including fever, coughing, and sore throats.

Another herb that has pungent anti-inflammatory, antioxidant, and immune-modulating qualities that may be helpful in combating new viral threats is turmeric (Curcuma longa). Turmeric's primary active ingredient, curcumin, has been demonstrated to enhance immune function, lessen inflammation, and halt the spread of infections. Research has indicated that taking a turmeric supplement may lessen the intensity and length of symptoms experienced by those infected with viruses. It may also help avert consequences like pneumonia and acute respiratory distress syndrome (ARDS).

The traditional Chinese herb Astragalus, also known as Astragalus membranaceus, is prized for its antiviral and immune-boosting qualities. It has been demonstrated that the polysaccharides, flavonoids, and saponins found in Astragalus improve immune system performance, boost the formation of white blood cells, and prevent virus reproduction. Astragalus supplements have been shown in studies to reduce the severity and also duration of viral infections, including influenza as well as respiratory syncytial virus (RSV), in addition to aiding in the defense against infections that may cause bronchitis and pneumonia.

The possible antiviral activities of olive leaf extract (Olea europaea) have also been explored in herbal remedies.

Oleuropein, a substance found in olive leaf extract, has been demonstrated to impede viral replication by preventing viral attachment to and entry into host cells. Research has indicated that the administration of supplements containing olive leaf extract may lessen the intensity and length of symptoms experienced by people infected with viruses such as the influenza virus, herpes simplex virus (HSV), and human immunodeficiency virus (HIV). It may also help avert complications like pneumonia and encephalitis.

Although using herbal medicines in conjunction with conventional medical care can be beneficial in treating growing virus risks, caution must be exercised when using them. Herbal medicine is a valuable tool to improve immune function, relieve symptoms, and enhance general well-being. It should not be used in place of antiviral drugs, vaccines, or other prescription therapies. To guarantee the safe and efficient use of medicinal herbs, it's also crucial to speak with a trained healthcare provider before beginning any herbal cure, especially if you're taking medicine or have any underlying medical conditions. Herbal remedies for new viral threats can be helpful instruments for improving resistance and lessening the effect of infectious diseases on world health if used carefully and with concern for safety.

CHAPTER V

Integrating Herbal Practices into Daily Life

Herbal Immune Support

For ages, herbal immune support has been a fundamental component of traditional medical systems. A wide range of herbs are known to bolster the body's inherent defenses against illnesses and infections. Scientific studies have provided more evidence in recent years supporting the effectiveness of several of these plants, illuminating their modes of action and possible medical advantages. A vast array of botanicals, each with its own distinct set of bioactive chemicals that have antibacterial, anti-inflammatory, and immunomodulatory properties, are included in the category of herbal immune support.

Probably one of the most well-known and thoroughly studied herbs for immune support is echinacea (Echinacea purpurea). Echinacea, a native of North America, has long been used traditionally by Indigenous peoples for its capacity to strengthen immunity and advance general health. Several bioactive substances, such as polysaccharides, alkamides, and flavonoids, have been found in echinacea in contemporary studies. These substances have been demonstrated to boost the body's defenses against infections, promote immune cell activity, and raise cytokine synthesis. Clinical research has shown that taking echinacea supplements can lessen the intensity and also the length of respiratory infections, such as the flu and the common cold, and when taken preventively, may also help avoid repeated infections.

Elderberry (Sambucus nigra), another well-liked herb for immune support, is well-known for its abundance of flavonoids, anthocyanins, and antioxidants. Because of the antiviral and immune-stimulating qualities of elderberries, they have a long history of traditional use in both Europe and North America. Studies have demonstrated that extracts from elderberries can prevent the growth of certain viruses, such as the herpes simplex virus (HSV) and influenza, and they may also lessen the intensity and length of respiratory illnesses. Supplementing with elderberries has been linked to improved immune cell function, higher cytokine production, and alleviation of symptoms in people suffering from the flu, the common cold, and other viral infections.

Astragalus (Astragalus membranaceus), a common herb in traditional Chinese medicine (TCM), is highly valued for its immune-stimulating and adaptogenic properties. Polysaccharides, flavonoids, and saponins found in astragalus have been demonstrated to strengthen the immune system, boost the generation of white blood cells, and help the body adjust to stressful situations. Supplementing with astragalus has been shown in studies to lessen the incidence and intensity of respiratory infections, including the flu and colds, as well as to help perhaps avoid consequences like pneumonia. Often used as a tonic herb, astragalus promotes general energy and resistance to disease.

The adaptable herb ginger (Zingiber officinale) has been utilized for millennia in traditional medical systems all throughout the world because of its immune-boosting qualities. Bioactive substances found in ginger, such as shogaol and gingerol, have been demonstrated to have antibacterial, anti-inflammatory, and antioxidant properties. According to studies, eating supplements containing ginger can boost immunity, reduce inflammation, and lessen the symptoms of respiratory infections, such as coughing, sore throats, and congestion. Ginger tea is a calming medicine that is frequently used to strengthen immune function and enhance respiratory well-being. It is created by steeping fresh ginger slices in hot water.

Another plant with strong immune-modulating and anti-inflammatory qualities that have drawn interest due to its possible health benefits is turmeric (Curcuma longa). Turmeric's primary active component, curcumin, has been demonstrated to improve the body's defenses against infections, lessen inflammatory reactions, and alter immune cell function.

Studies have indicated that taking a turmeric supplement may lessen the intensity and length of respiratory infections, such as the flu and colds, as well as aid with the symptoms of inflammatory illnesses like autoimmune diseases and arthritis. Turmeric is widely used as a spice in food preparation and as a medicinal herb. It comes in many different forms, including teas, pills, and extracts.

Traditional medical systems have utilized licorice root (Glycyrrhiza glabra), a therapeutic herb with immune-modulating and antiviral qualities, for millennia. Glycyrrhizin, a substance found in licorice root, has been demonstrated to increase immune cell activity, prevent virus replication, and lessen inflammation. Taking supplements containing licorice root can improve immunity, lessen the intensity and length of respiratory infections, and possibly even help avoid consequences like pneumonia. Herbal remedies for respiratory health and immunological support frequently include licorice root.

Although using herbal immune support therapies in conjunction with other supporting measures can be good for boosting general health and well-being, caution must be exercised when using them. Getting adequate sleep, drinking plenty of water, eating a balanced diet, controlling stress, and maintaining good hygiene are all critical for maintaining a robust immune system and also reducing the risk of infections. It's also essential to see a qualified healthcare professional before starting any herbal therapy, especially if you have any underlying medical conditions or are on medication, to ensure the safe and effective use of medicinal herbs. Herbal immune support can be a valuable tool for promoting optimal health and wellness and boosting resilience when used correctly and with attention to safety precautions.

Herbal Remedies for Prevention

The ability of herbal treatments to promote general health and lower the risk of illness and disease has long been recognized as a valuable preventive measure. Herbalism, which has its roots in ancient medical practices from all over the world, provides a plethora of botanicals with antibacterial, antioxidant, and immune-boosting qualities. These herbs can be included in everyday routines to support resilience against various health concerns and bolster the body's natural defenses.

One of the most well-known herbs for immune support and protection is echinacea (Echinacea purpurea). Echinacea is a native of North America, and Indigenous peoples have been using it for generations to boost immunity and prevent illnesses. Several bioactive substances, such as polysaccharides, alkamides, and flavonoids, have been found in echinacea in contemporary studies. These substances boost immune cell function and improve the body's defenses against infections.

Supplementing with echinacea has been linked to a decreased incidence of upper respiratory infections, which include the flu and the common cold, as well as shorter sickness duration and milder symptoms when the disease does strike.

Elderberry (Sambucus nigra), another herb well-known for its prophylactic qualities, is rich in antioxidants, flavonoids, and anthocyanins. Elderberries have long been used traditionally in Europe and North America due to their immune-stimulating and antiviral properties. Studies have demonstrated that extracts from elderberries can prevent the growth of certain viruses, such as the herpes simplex virus (HSV) and influenza, and they may also lessen the intensity and length of respiratory illnesses. Including elderberry in regular wellness practices, like drinking elderberry tea or syrup, can boost immunity and lower the chance of infection.

Popular in traditional Chinese medicine (TCM), astragalus (Astragalus membranaceus) is prized for its immune-stimulating and adaptogenic qualities. Polysaccharides, flavonoids, and saponins found in astragalus have been demonstrated to strengthen the immune system, boost the generation of white blood cells, and help the body adjust to stressful situations. Frequent use of astragalus tea or tincture can enhance general vigor and resistance to sickness, lowering the risk of infections and encouraging a quicker recovery in the event that sickness does strike.

Allium sativum, or garlic, is a culinary and medicinal herb that has strong antibacterial and immune-stimulating qualities. Allicin, one of the sulfur-containing chemicals found in garlic, has been demonstrated to both enhance immune cell activity and impede the growth of bacteria, viruses, and fungi. Regular garlic consumption has been shown to lower blood pressure and also cholesterol levels, as well as the risk of upper respiratory infections like the flu and colds. Adding garlic to meals on a regular basis or supplementing with garlic can boost immunity and promote general health.

Another herb with strong preventative qualities is turmeric (Curcuma longa), which has anti-inflammatory, antioxidant, and immune-modulating qualities. It has been shown that curcumin, the main active component of turmeric, influences immune cell function, reduces inflammation, and strengthens the body's defenses against infections. According to studies, taking supplements containing turmeric may lower inflammation and oxidative stress, which in turn may reduce the likelihood of contracting long-term conditions such as Alzheimer's disease, cancer, and heart disease. Turmeric pills or meal additions can boost immune system performance and offer protection against numerous health risks.

Zingiber officinale, or ginger, is a multipurpose herb that has immune-stimulating and antibacterial qualities that make it useful for prevention. Bioactive substances found in ginger, such as shogaol and gingerol, have been demonstrated to promote immune cell activity and impede the growth of germs and viruses. Regular consumption of ginger has been shown in studies to help relieve the symptoms of gastrointestinal illnesses and arthritis, as well as lower the risk of infections like the flu and colds. Blending ginger into drinks, smoothies, or meals can boost immunity and improve general health.

Glycyrrhiza glabra, or licorice root, is a medicinal herb that has antiviral and immune-modulating qualities that make it useful for prophylaxis. Glycyrrhizin, a substance found in licorice root, has been demonstrated to increase immune cell activity, prevent virus replication, and lessen inflammation. Studies have shown that taking licorice root on a daily basis can help lower the incidence of upper respiratory infections and relieve allergies and gastrointestinal issues. Licorice root may be used as a supplement, tincture, or tea to promote general health and immune system function.

Herbal medicines are helpful tools for prevention, but it's crucial to utilize them in conjunction with other holistic wellness practices. A robust immune system and lower risk of illness depend on a balanced diet, frequent exercise, stress reduction, and good cleanliness habits. To guarantee the safe and efficient use of medicinal herbs, it's also crucial to speak with a trained healthcare provider before beginning any herbal cure, especially if you're taking medicine or have any underlying medical conditions. Herbal medicines have the potential to improve immune function and promote optimal health and well-being when used with caution and with consideration for preventive actions.

Herbal Treatments for Acute Infections

Herbal remedies for acute infections provide a safe, all-natural method of symptom management, immune system support, and healing. Common illnesses known as acute infections, which can cause discomfort and interfere with everyday life, include colds, the flu, sinus infections, and urinary tract infections. Herbal medicine provides a complementary approach that can help relieve symptoms, reduce inflammation, and strengthen the body's natural defenses against infections. At the same time, conventional medical treatments concentrate on treating the symptoms and using antibiotics or antiviral drugs to target the underlying cause.

One of the most well-known and thoroughly studied herbs for acute infections is echinacea (Echinacea purpurea). Echinacea is a native of North America, and Indigenous peoples have been using it for generations to stimulate their immune systems. Several bioactive substances, such as polysaccharides, alkamides, and flavonoids, have been found in echinacea in contemporary studies. These substances have been demonstrated to improve immune function and lessen the intensity and duration of respiratory illnesses, such as the flu and the common cold. When symptoms first appear, echinacea tinctures or supplements are frequently taken to boost immune system activity and encourage a quicker recovery.

Another herb that has antiviral solid and immune-stimulating qualities that can be utilized for acute infections is elderberry (Sambucus nigra). Elderberries have long been used traditionally in North America and Europe to treat respiratory illnesses such as colds and the flu by lessening their intensity and duration. Elderberry extracts have been demonstrated in studies to prevent the growth of certain viruses, such as the herpes simplex virus (HSV) and the influenza virus. They may also be able to reduce symptoms, including fever, coughing, and congestion. Lozenges or syrup made from elderberries are common treatments for acute respiratory infections.

Acute infections can benefit from the use of garlic (Allium sativum), a culinary and medicinal herb with antibacterial, antiviral, and immune-boosting qualities. Allicin, one of the sulfur-containing chemicals found in garlic, has been demonstrated to both enhance immune cell activity and impede the growth of bacteria, viruses, and fungi. Studies have indicated that taking supplements containing garlic may help lower blood pressure and cholesterol, as well as lessen the intensity and length of colds, the flu, and other respiratory illnesses. When symptoms appear, use raw garlic or supplements containing garlic to boost immunity and expedite healing.

A multipurpose herb that can be used for acute infections, ginger (Zingiber officinale) has antibacterial, anti-inflammatory, and immune-boosting qualities. Bioactive substances found in ginger, such as shogaol and gingerol, have been demonstrated to lower inflammation and also stop the growth of germs and viruses. Studies have shown that taking supplements containing ginger can help reduce the symptoms of gastrointestinal issues, arthritis, and respiratory infections, including cough, sore throat, and congestion. During acute infections, consistent consumption of ginger tea or ginger capsules can improve immune function and promote overall well-beingwell-being.

Acute infections can benefit from the usage of licorice root (Glycyrrhiza glabra), a medicinal herb with immune-modulating and antiviral qualities. Glycyrrhizin, a substance found in licorice root, has been demonstrated to increase immune cell activity, prevent virus replication, and lessen inflammation. Studies have shown that taking supplements containing licorice root helps lessen the intensity and length of colds, the flu, and other respiratory illnesses. It can also help ease the symptoms of allergies and gastrointestinal issues. To boost immune function and hasten recovery from acute infections, drink licorice root tea or licorice supplements.

Another herb that can be used for acute infections is turmeric (Curcuma longa), which has potent anti-inflammatory, antioxidant, and immune-boosting qualities. Studies have indicated that taking a turmeric supplement may lessen the intensity and length of colds, the flu, and other respiratory infections. It can also help improve the symptoms of inflammatory illnesses like autoimmune diseases and arthritis. During acute illnesses, taking turmeric tea or capsules on a regular basis boosts immunity and improves general health.

Herbal remedies for acute infections have the potential to reduce symptoms and speed up healing, but they should only be used sparingly and in concert with other supportive therapies. Managing acute infections and lowering the risk of consequences requires enough rest, water, nutrition, and adherence to appropriate hygiene measures. To guarantee the safe and efficient use of medicinal herbs, it's also crucial to speak with a trained healthcare provider before beginning any herbal cure, especially if you're taking medicine or have any underlying medical conditions. Herbal remedies for acute infections can be helpful instruments for fostering the best possible health and well-being if they are used with caution and consideration for preventative measures.

Long-term Management Strategies

For those who are dealing with persistent health issues or chronic medical illnesses, long-term treatment techniques are crucial. These tactics comprise a thorough approach to treatment that attends to the condition's underlying causes, risk factors, and possible complications in addition to its symptoms. Adopting appropriate management measures can greatly enhance quality of life and increase overall well-being, whether negotiating the challenges of long-term rehabilitation from a catastrophic injury or illness, or managing a chronic illness such as diabetes, hypertension, or autoimmune disease.

Modifying one's lifestyle is a crucial part of long-term management measures. Optimizing health outcomes and lowering the risk of problems related to chronic illnesses can be achieved by implementing good lifestyle habits such regular exercise, a balanced diet, stress management, getting enough sleep, and abstaining from dangerous substances. Particularly, physical activity has been demonstrated to offer a host of advantages for both mental and physical health, such as greater immune system performance, decreased inflammation, enhanced cardiovascular health, and improved mood regulation. Walking, swimming, or yoga are examples of regular exercise that can be incorporated into everyday routines to assist people manage their disease and preserve general health and mobility.

Medication management is a crucial component of long-term care. Following recommended treatment plans and keeping an eye on medication use are essential for attaining the best possible health results for people with chronic diseases that call for continued medication. This could entail carefully collaborating with medical professionals to guarantee that prescriptions are taken as prescribed, keeping an eye out for any possible interactions or adverse effects, and modifying treatment plans as necessary. Furthermore, techniques like pill organizers, medication reminders, and medication reviews can enhance adherence and lower the chance of medication errors for those with complicated drug schedules.

Regular monitoring and follow-up treatment are common components of long-term management techniques, in addition to drug management and lifestyle modification. This can entail regular check-ups with medical professionals, tracking of important health indicators like weight, blood pressure, blood sugar, and cholesterol, and recurring evaluations of the success of treatment or the advancement of the condition. Frequent monitoring makes it possible to identify changes in health status early and to take prompt action to manage or prevent consequences. Additionally, it offers chances for continued instruction and assistance to help people comprehend their situation and make wise health-related judgments.

Self-management and self-care are crucial components of long-term management. Better outcomes and a greater standard of living can arise from providing people with the resources they need to actively manage their own health and wellness. This could entail picking up self-care skills for handling symptoms or flare-ups, as well as self-management measures like stress reduction, symptom monitoring, and relaxation techniques. It may also require dietary adjustments, frequent exercise, and the acquisition of stress-reduction techniques in order to enhance the treatment of the condition and reduce the likelihood of complications.

Long-term management options may include complementary and alternative therapies in addition to medication management, self-care, lifestyle adjustment, and routine monitoring to support general health and well-being. These could include therapies like massage therapy, herbal medicine, acupuncture, chiropractic adjustments, and mind-body exercises like tai chi, yoga, and meditation. These therapies can supplement traditional medical care while not replacing it. They can offer extra assistance for symptom management, stress reduction, and quality of life enhancement.

All things considered, long-term management techniques are critical to fostering the best possible health and wellbeing in people with chronic illnesses or persistent health issues. Individuals can effectively manage their disease, lower their risk of problems, and enhance their overall quality of life by implementing complementary therapies, monitoring their health, practicing self-care, and adopting good lifestyle practices. A proactive approach to care and strong collaboration with healthcare practitioners can help people meet their health objectives and successfully manage the challenges of long-term care.

CHAPTER VI

Case Studies and Success Stories

Personal Experiences with Herbal Antiviral Practices
Firsthand accounts of herbal antiviral treatments provide essential information about the efficacy, safety, and general effects of utilizing medicinal herbs to treat viral infections. Anecdotal evidence from personal experiences can supplement and deepen our understanding of herbal medicines, even while scientific research offers significant proof of their usefulness. Personal stories can provide insight into the variety of applications of herbal medicine in everyday life, from treating ordinary colds and flu to more severe viral disorders like herpes and lung infections.

Many people first turn to herbal antiviral techniques in an attempt to treat common respiratory illnesses like the flu or the common cold. People may use herbal medicines like echinacea, elderberry, ginger, and garlic to assist in relieving symptoms and support immune function when symptoms like sore throat, congestion, and exhaustion appear. These remedies can be used either on their own or in conjunction with other natural therapies or conventional treatments. They can be consumed in a variety of formats, such as teas, tinctures, capsules, or handmade remedies. Anecdotal evidence frequently emphasizes the speedy beginning of alleviation and amelioration of symptoms following the use of herbal treatments, along with the general sense of well-being and vigor that is regained during the healing process.

Personal experiences with herbal antiviral techniques may encompass treating persistent viral illnesses like herpes simplex virus (HSV) in addition to acute respiratory infections. Herpes is a widespread viral infection that can result in cold sores or genital herpes outbreaks, causing discomfort, humiliation, and mental anguish in those who have it. While antiviral drugs like acyclovir or valacyclovir are the standard treatments for herpes, some people find relief with natural therapies like lemon balm, licorice root, or tea tree oil. Anecdotes from personal experience frequently demonstrate how well these treatments work in lessening the frequency and intensity of herpes outbreaks, as well as the general improvement in quality of life and emotional health that many with this chronic illness experience.

Individuals may also benefit from using herbal antiviral remedies to treat more severe viral illnesses like influenza or respiratory syncytial virus (RSV). Despite the serious health dangers associated with these illnesses, particularly for small children, the elderly, and those with weakened immune systems, herbal therapies may be an adjunct to traditional medical care. Anecdotes from personal experience may emphasize the use of herbs to improve immune function, reduce inflammation, and aid in the healing process from respiratory infections, such as astragalus, licorice root, or olive leaf extract. People might talk about how they have used herbal medicines in addition to prescription drugs or other supporting therapies and how this has helped them achieve great results and reduce their symptoms.

The variety of viewpoints and methods that people apply while using medicinal herbs is one of the benefits of firsthand encounters with herbal antiviral therapies. Some people may use herbal treatments only to treat viral infections. Still, others may incorporate herbs into a more comprehensive wellness program that also includes dietary adjustments, lifestyle modifications, and other complementary therapies. Personal accounts may also emphasize the value of seeking advice on the safe and efficient use of herbal treatments from licensed healthcare providers, such as naturopathic physicians or herbalists. By contributing their experiences, people can broaden the body of information and help others understand the potential benefits of herbal antiviral remedies for their own health journey.

Finally, firsthand accounts of the effectiveness of herbal antiviral treatments provide essential context for understanding the variety of methods that medicinal herbs are employed to treat viral infections. Personal stories offer anecdotal evidence to scientific studies on the safety and efficiency of herbal medicines, covering a range of ailments from common colds and flu to chronic illnesses like herpes and respiratory infections. People who share their experiences help to advance knowledge of the advantages, difficulties, and subtleties of applying herbal therapy in practical contexts. By means of transparent communication, teamwork, and well-informed decision-making, people can effectively utilize herbal antiviral treatments to bolster their overall health and wellness.

Testimonials from Practitioners and Patients

Insights into the effectiveness, safety, and overall influence of herbal antiviral techniques in clinical settings and real-world experiences are greatly enhanced by the testimonies of practitioners and patients. For millennia, herbal medicine has been a fundamental component of healthcare systems worldwide, providing plant-based natural medicines that promote health and well-being. Testimonials give anecdotal information that can supplement and deepen our understanding of herbal medicines, even while scientific research offers significant proof of their efficacy. Testimonials from naturopathic physicians and herbalists to people in charge of their own health show the variety of applications and experiences with herbal antiviral therapies.

Herbalists, naturopathic physicians, and traditional healers are among the practitioners of herbal medicine who frequently offer case studies from their clinical practice to demonstrate the efficacy of herbal medicines in treating viral infections. Case studies, patient tales, and clinical observations that demonstrate the benefits of herbal medicine in boosting immunity, lowering viral loads, and enhancing general health may be included in these testimonies. Practitioners can discuss how they have treated more severe illnesses like respiratory syncytial virus (RSV) or human immunodeficiency virus (HIV), as well as common viral infections like the cold, flu, or herpes using certain herbs or herbal formulations. Through their experiences, practitioners add to the increasing amount of data that backs up the application of herbal antiviral treatments in clinical settings.

Patients who have personally benefited from herbal antiviral methods frequently share their experiences in order to encourage others and give hope to those who are dealing with comparable health issues. These testimonies could come from people who have used herbal remedies—alone or in conjunction with conventional treatments—to successfully manage viral infections. Patients can discuss how they have used particular herbs, herbal remedies, or dietary supplements to reduce symptoms, strengthen their immune systems, and aid in their general recovery from viral infections. They might also stress the value of individualized treatment, teamwork with medical professionals, and the sense of empowerment that results from actively participating in one's own health and well-being. Patients who share their tales might encourage those looking for alternative methods of health and recovery, as well as provide insightful information about the practical effects of herbal antiviral therapies.

Patient and practitioner testimonials can provide insight into the various ways that herbal antiviral techniques are incorporated into holistic medical approaches. They might emphasize the value of customized treatment programs made to fit the particular requirements, preferences, and health objectives of every individual. Testimonials may also stress how crucial it is to use herbal treatments with knowledge, communication, and sound judgment, particularly for those managing complicated or chronic medical conditions. Practitioners and patients add to a community body of knowledge by sharing their experiences, educating, and enabling others to investigate the possible advantages of herbal antiviral techniques in their own health journeys.

Testimonials may address common questions or misconceptions regarding herbal medication, such as safety, efficacy, and accessibility, in addition to stressing the advantages of herbal antiviral therapies. Patients and practitioners can exchange stories on utilizing herbs sensibly and safely, seeking advice from licensed medical professionals, and incorporating herbal treatments into all-encompassing treatment regimens. To guarantee consistency and efficacy, they can also go over the significance of quality control, standardized dosage, and trustworthy suppliers of herbal goods. Testimonials assist in demystifying herbal medicine and increase its accessibility for people looking for alternative methods of health and healing by addressing these issues.

Finally, testimonies from healthcare professionals and patients offer insightful information about the effectiveness, safety, and overall impact of herbal antiviral practices in real-world situations and clinical settings. Practitioners and patients alike are adding to the expanding body of evidence supporting the use of herbal treatments for controlling viral infections and enhancing general health and well-being by sharing their own tales.

Their testimonies provide others hope, support, and the confidence to investigate the potential advantages of herbal antiviral treatments in their own health journeys. By means of transparent communication, teamwork, and well-informed decision-making, people can effectively utilize herbal medicine to enhance their overall health and wellness.

Real-life Applications of Herbal Solutions

Herbal remedies may be used in a variety of real-world situations within the framework of herbal antiviral techniques. These include treating viral illnesses ranging from herpes to respiratory syncytial virus (RSV), HIV, and common colds and flu. Rooted in ancient medical systems worldwide, herbal medicine provides a wide range of plant-based medicines that have been used for millennia to enhance general wellness, relieve symptoms, and boost the immune system. While empirical studies offer valuable proof of the effectiveness of herbal medicines, real-world applications provide firsthand accounts that emphasize the usefulness, efficacy, and adaptability of herbal antiviral therapies in daily life.

Herbal remedies are frequently used in real life to treat acute respiratory illnesses like the flu and the common cold. People may use herbal medicines, including echinacea, elderberry, ginger, and garlic, as soon as symptoms appear in order to help reduce symptoms and boost immunity. These remedies can be used either on their own or in conjunction with other natural therapies or conventional treatments. They can be consumed in a variety of formats, such as teas, tinctures, capsules, or handmade remedies. Experiences from actual patients frequently attest to the quick onset of alleviation and improvement in symptoms following the use of herbal treatments, as well as the general sense of well-being and vigor that is restored during the healing process.

Herbal remedies are utilized not just to treat acute respiratory infections but also to treat chronic viral illnesses like herpes simplex virus (HSV). Herpes is a common virus that can produce outbreaks of genital herpes or cold sores, causing discomfort and psychological misery in those who have it. While antiviral drugs like acyclovir or valacyclovir are the standard treatments for herpes, some people find relief with natural therapies like lemon balm, licorice root, or tea tree oil. Experiences from real-world situations frequently demonstrate how well these treatments work to lessen the frequency and intensity of herpes outbreaks as well as the general improvement in quality of life and emotional health that those with this chronic illness report.

Treating more severe viral illnesses like the human immunodeficiency virus (HIV) and respiratory syncytial virus (RSV) in real life is another use for herbal remedies. Despite the severe health dangers associated with these illnesses, particularly for small children, the elderly, and those with weakened immune systems, herbal therapies may be an adjunct to traditional medical care. Herbs like astragalus, licorice root, or olive leaf extract have been used in real life to boost immunity, lower inflammation, and speed up the healing process after respiratory infections. People might talk about how they have used herbal medicines in addition to prescription drugs or other supporting therapies and how this has helped them achieve great results and reduce their symptoms.

Herbal remedies have real-world uses that go beyond curing particular viral infections to promote general health and wellness. Herbal medicines have the potential to enhance immune function, decrease inflammation, and facilitate the body's inherent healing mechanisms when integrated into regular routines. Herbs like echinacea, ginger, turmeric, and garlic can be used by people as preventative measures to lower their risk of illness and enhance their general health. Using these herbs in food preparation, preparing herbal tinctures or teas, or consuming herbal supplements as part of a holistic health routine are examples of real-world applications.

Overall, the practicality, efficacy, and adaptability of herbal antiviral techniques in daily life are demonstrated by real-world uses of herbal treatments. Herbal treatments offer a natural and holistic approach to strengthening immune function, relieving symptoms, and improving quality of life. They can be used to manage acute respiratory infections and chronic viral illnesses and support general health and wellness. People add to a growing body of knowledge by sharing their experiences, which enlightens and encourages others to investigate the possible advantages of herbal antiviral treatments in their own health journey. People can use herbal medicine to improve their health and vitality in practical ways by having open discussions, working together, and making well-informed decisions.

CHAPTER VII. Herbal Medicine and Holistic Health

The Mind-Body Connection in Healing

A key idea in holistic health and herbal medicine, the mind-body link emphasizes the complex interrelationships between mental, emotional, and physical well-being. Holistic health techniques, which have their roots in age-old healing practices from all over the world, acknowledge the connection and mutual effect of the mind and body. Integrative health practices' mainstay, herbal medicine, uses plants' healing properties to enhance the body's natural ability to heal itself and advance general well-being. Herbal medicine practitioners and those looking for holistic health solutions can maximize health outcomes and improve quality of life by comprehending and fostering the mind-body link.

Understanding that our ideas, feelings, beliefs, and attitudes may have a significant impact on our physical health and well-being is fundamental to the mind-body link in healing. It has been demonstrated that stress, anxiety, sadness, and other negative emotions impair immunity, raise inflammatory levels, and aid in the onset and advancement of chronic illnesses. Positive emotions, on the other hand, such as happiness, appreciation, and optimism, have been connected to better overall health outcomes, decreased inflammation, and enhanced immune function. Herbal therapy promotes healing on all levels of being by addressing the underlying emotional and energetic imbalances that lead to sickness through the use of plant-based treatments.

Herbal therapy addresses the underlying emotional and spiritual factors that affect health in addition to the physical symptoms of illness, therefore promoting the mind-body connection. Due to their adaptogenic qualities, many herbs used in holistic health practices aid in the body's ability to adjust to stress and stabilize the nervous system. Adaptogens that enhance stress resilience, balance cortisol levels, and promote general well-being include rhodiola, holy basil, and ashwagandha. Herbal treatments support deep, comprehensive healing by addressing the underlying causes of illness and fostering harmony and balance within the body.

Herbal medicine promotes the mind-body link by addressing emotional and energy imbalances and emphasizing individualized, patient-centered therapy. Herbalists and holistic health professionals consider an individual's particular constitution, lifestyle, surroundings, and spiritual beliefs in addition to the physical symptoms of their condition. Herbal therapy respects the body's innate ability to cure itself and recognizes the interdependence of mind, body, and spirit by treating the whole individual rather than simply the disease's symptoms. Through the development of a sense of empowerment, autonomy, and self-awareness, this patient-centered approach enables people to participate actively in their own recovery process.

Herbal medicine approaches frequently include mind-body techniques, such as mindfulness, meditation, visualization, and breathwork, to augment the healing process and foster general wellness. By lowering tension, worry, and other unpleasant feelings that can compromise one's health and well-being, these methods assist people in developing a condition of inner harmony and balance. Mind-body techniques enhance the therapeutic benefits of herbal treatments by fostering calm, decreasing inflammation, and bolstering the immune system, thus fostering a synergistic approach to holistic recovery. Herbal medicine encourages a closer bond with nature and the natural world, which further bolsters the mind-body connection. Many herbal treatments come from plants that indigenous civilizations have been using for their medical qualities for generations. People can access a plentiful supply of restorative energy and vigor by reestablishing a connection with the natural world and the wisdom of conventional treatment methods. A greater understanding of the interdependence of all living things and the significance of coexisting peacefully with nature for one's health and well-being is fostered by herbal treatment.

In summary, the mind-body link emphasizes the interdependence of mental, emotional, and physical health and is a fundamental idea in holistic health and herbal medicine. Herbal medicine addresses the underlying mental and energetic imbalances that contribute to sickness, providing a holistic approach to healing that promotes the mind-body connection. Herbal medicines enhance the body's natural ability to repair itself and promote general well-being by fostering balance, harmony, and resilience on all levels of being. This allows for profound, holistic healing. Herbal medicine encourages people to actively participate in their own healing process by emphasizing individualized, patient-centered care and mind-body practices like mindfulness, meditation, and visualization. This promotes a sense of empowerment, autonomy, and self-awareness that supports long-term health and vitality.

Herbal Practices for Emotional Well-being

The profound interplay between mental, emotional, and physical well-being is highlighted by the mind-body connection, which is a basic idea in holistic health and herbal therapy. Holistic health approaches, originating from historic therapeutic traditions worldwide, acknowledge the interdependence of the mind and body and their mutual influence on one another's physiological functioning. A fundamental component of holistic health care, herbal medicine uses the therapeutic properties of plants to assist the body's natural ability to repair itself and to advance general well-being. By recognizing and promoting the mind-body connection, holistic health seekers and herbal medicine practitioners may improve their overall quality of life and optimize their health outcomes.

Realizing how much our ideas, feelings, beliefs, and attitudes may affect our physical health and well-being is fundamental to the mind-body link in healing. It has been demonstrated that negative emotions such as stress, worry, and sadness impair immunity, raise inflammation, and aid in the onset and advancement of chronic illnesses.

On the other hand, happy, thankful, and optimistic feelings have been connected to better overall health outcomes, decreased inflammation, and enhanced immune system performance. By utilizing plant-based medicines, herbal therapy promotes healing on all levels of being by providing a comprehensive approach to resolving the underlying emotional and energetic imbalances that lead to sickness.

By treating the underlying emotional and spiritual factors that affect health in addition to the outward signs of disease, herbal medicine promotes the mind-body link. Numerous herbs utilized in holistic health methods include adaptogenic qualities, which enable the body to adjust to stress and reestablish nervous system homeostasis. Adaptogens, which include Rhodiola, holy basil, and ashwagandha, can help control cortisol levels, increase stress tolerance, and promote general well-being. Herbal treatments enhance healing on a profound, comprehensive level by addressing the underlying causes of illness and fostering balance and harmony within the body.

Herbal medicine not only treats emotional and energy imbalances but also promotes the mind-body connection by emphasizing individualized, patient-centered therapy. In addition to considering an individual's particular constitution, lifestyle, surroundings, and spiritual beliefs, herbalists and holistic health practitioners also consider the physical signs of illness. Herbal therapy recognizes the interdependence of mind, body, and spirit and respects the body's innate ability to cure itself by treating the whole individual rather than just the disease's symptoms. This patient-centered approach helps people develop a sense of agency, self-awareness, and empowerment so they can actively participate in their own healing process.

Herbal medicine approaches frequently include mind-body practices like mindfulness, meditation, visualization, and breathwork to support general wellness and speed up the healing process. These methods assist people in developing a condition of inner harmony and balance while lowering tension, worry, and other unfavorable feelings that may compromise their health and general well-being. Herbal medicines have therapeutic effects, but mind-body techniques enhance them by boosting immunity, lowering inflammation, and encouraging relaxation. This results in a synergistic approach to holistic health.

By encouraging a closer bond with nature and the natural world, herbal medicine also contributes to the mind-body connection. Numerous herbal medicines are made from plants that native cultures have been using for their therapeutic qualities for generations. People can access a plentiful supply of healing energy and vitality by reestablishing a connection with the natural world and by acquiring knowledge of conventional treatment methods.

Herbal medicine helps people get a greater understanding of how all living things are interconnected and how important it is to live in harmony with the natural world in order to live as healthily and well as possible.

To sum up, the mind-body link is a fundamental idea in herbal medicine and holistic health that highlights the connection between mental, emotional, and physical wellness. By treating the underlying mental and energetic imbalances that contribute to illness, herbal medicine provides a comprehensive approach to healing that promotes the mind-body connection. Herbal treatments support deep, holistic healing by fostering resilience, harmony, and balance on all levels of being. This enhances the body's natural ability to heal itself and advances general wellness. Herbal medicine fosters a sense of empowerment, autonomy, and self-awareness that supports lifelong health and vitality by emphasizing personalized, patient-centered care and mind-body techniques like mindfulness, meditation, and visualization. This allows people to participate actively in their own healing process.

Lifestyle Factors and Herbal Support

Integrative health practices are built on lifestyle factors, which are critical in establishing overall health and well-being and which are bolstered by herbal assistance. With its roots in age-old healing practices from all over the world, herbal medicine acknowledges the connection between lifestyle decisions and how they affect one's physical, mental, and emotional well-being. Herbal medicine practitioners and others looking for holistic health solutions can maximize health outcomes and promote wellness on all levels of being by addressing lifestyle aspects like nutrition, exercise, stress management, sleep hygiene, and social relationships.

One of the most basic lifestyle elements influencing health is diet, and herbal medicine provides a plethora of plant-based therapies to assist good digestion and nutrition. Numerous herbs are abundant in nutrients that support and nourish the body's essential organ systems, including vitamins, minerals, antioxidants, and phytonutrients. Herbs that help with digestion and ease gastrointestinal discomfort include ginger, peppermint, and fennel; they also assist liver health and detoxification when used in herbal medicines like dandelion root, burdock root, and milk thistle. People can enhance their overall health, vitamin absorption, and digestion by including nutrient-dense foods and herbal medicines in their diet.

Another crucial lifestyle component that enhances general health and well-being is exercise, and herbal medicine provides botanical treatments to stimulate physical activity and boost vitality—known as adaptogens, herbs like ashwagandha, Rhodiola, and ginseng support energy and endurance while assisting the body in adjusting to stress on both a physical and mental level. These herbs increase resilience and stamina, boost overall athletic performance, and promote the body's natural reaction to physical exertion. People can receive the advantages of consistent physical activity and maximize their physical fitness by adding adaptogenic herbs to their workout regimen.

Maintaining good health and well-being requires effective stress management, and herbal medicine provides a range of plant medicines to support emotional balance, lessen anxiety, and assist relaxation. Herbs with relaxing qualities that support relaxation and assist in calming the nervous system include chamomile, lavender, and lemon balm. Herbs known to be adaptogenic, such as Schisandra, holy basil, and reishi mushroom, aid in the body's ability to cope with stress and build resistance against illnesses brought on by it. People can build a sense of inner peace and tranquility, lessen the harmful effects of chronic stress, and promote general emotional well-being by including stress-reducing herbs in their daily routine.

Another significant lifestyle aspect that affects health is sleep hygiene. Herbal medicine provides botanical medicines that assist restful sleep and encourage ideal sleep patterns. Herbs with sedative qualities, such as passionflower, valerian, and hops, can help induce calm and encourage sound sleep. These herbs help the body's normal circadian rhythm, enhance the length and quality of sleep, and reduce insomnia and other sleep-related issues. People can increase the quality of their sleep, improve their sleep hygiene, and wake up feeling renewed by adding herbs that promote sleep to their nighttime regimen.

Herbal therapy provides plant medicines to boost emotional well-being and foster social ties, two more essential components of holistic health. Herbs with mood-balancing qualities, like kava kava, mimosa bark, and St. John's wort, can help reduce anxiety, depression, and other mood disorders. These herbs promote emotional fortitude, elevate mood and perspective, and strengthen interpersonal connections. Herbs that support mood can help people develop a sense of community, make meaningful connections with others, and enhance their emotional health on a daily basis.

To sum up, lifestyle factors, including nutrition, exercise, stress reduction, good sleep hygiene, and social support, are essential determinants of general health and well-being. These aspects, when paired with herbal assistance, constitute the basis of holistic health practices. Numerous plant-based therapies are available in herbal medicine to promote healthy eating, exercise, stress reduction, restful sleep, and mental health. People can maximize their lifestyle choices, enhance holistic well-being, and develop resilience, energy, and balance that support lifetime health and well-being by adding herbal treatments into their daily routine. Herbal medicine encourages people to take an active role in their own health journey and reap the rewards of a robust, meaningful life by emphasizing holistic approaches to health and wellness.

Herbal Medicine as Part of a Comprehensive Health Plan

Herbal medicine is an essential component of holistic health strategies because it provides natural solutions that enhance and complement other holistic health approaches. Herbal medicine, which has its roots in age-old therapeutic practices from many cultures, acknowledges the connection between the mind, body, and spirit in fostering health and well-being. Herbal remedies can be used in complete health plans to help people handle a variety of health issues and achieve optimal well-being on all levels of existence.

The fundamental tenet of herbal medicine is the conviction that, with the right encouragement and nutrition, the body has the inherent capacity to heal itself. Herbal medicines support essential organ systems and enhance general health by supplying vital nutrients, antioxidants, and phytochemicals that interfere with the body's natural healing processes. Herbal therapy offers a holistic approach to health that respects the interdependence of all elements of being, whether it is used to treat underlying imbalances, enhance immunological function, or alleviate symptoms.

Herbal medicine's adaptability to specific health demands and preferences is one of its main advantages. Herbal treatments can be customized to address specific health issues by taking into consideration lifestyle factors, age, gender, and underlying medical disorders. In order to develop individualized treatment regimens that incorporate herbal treatments with other holistic health practices, including diet, exercise, stress management, and spiritual wellness, herbalists and holistic health practitioners collaborate closely with patients. Herbal medicine promotes all-encompassing health regimens that address the physical, mental, emotional, and also spiritual elements of well-being by addressing the underlying causes of sickness and fostering balance and harmony within the body.

Additionally, herbal medicine provides a long-term preventive approach to health, assisting people in preserving their vitality and well-being. Numerous herbs promote the body's natural defenses and also help prevent infections by strengthening the immune system.

Through the everyday use of immune-supporting herbs, people can increase their resistance to disease and advance their general health. Additionally, before they become more significant health issues, herbal treatments can be taken proactively to address common health concerns, including stress, exhaustion, sleeplessness, digestive disorders, and hormone imbalances. People can improve their quality of life and lower their risk of illness by adopting a proactive attitude to health and well-being.

Herbal treatments not only provide therapeutic benefits but also provide many people with a mild and safe substitute for conventional pharmaceuticals. Herbal therapy places a strong emphasis on using natural components and complete plant extracts to reduce the possibility of adverse side effects and drug interactions.

Herbal medicines can be safely used in conjunction with conventional treatments to increase their efficacy and lessen their adverse effects. They are frequently well-tolerated by people of all ages. People can access a wide choice of natural medicines that promote healing and well-being without the adverse effects of synthetic pharmaceuticals by incorporating herbal medicine into complete health regimens.

Herbal medicine also fosters a strong bond with the natural world and the natural world, as well as a sense of gratitude, reverence, and oneness with all living things. Many herbal treatments come from plants that indigenous civilizations have been using for their medical qualities for generations. People can access a plentiful supply of restorative energy and vigor by reestablishing a connection with the natural world and the wisdom of conventional treatment methods. In order to promote health and well-being, herbal medicine urges people to develop a deeper understanding of their relationship to the environment and to honor the interconnectedness of all living things.

In summary, herbal medicine is essential to all-encompassing health regimens since it provides natural solutions that enhance and supplement holistic medical approaches. Herbal remedies can be used in complete health plans to help people handle a variety of health issues and achieve optimal well-being on all levels of existence. Herbal medicine may offer a holistic approach to health that respects the interconnection of mind, body, and spirit. It can be used to relieve symptoms, improve immune function, prevent illness, or promote general wellness. Herbal medicine fosters a sense of balance, vitality, and wholeness that supports lifelong well-being and enables people to actively participate in their own health and well-being because of its adaptability, safety, and connection to nature.

CHAPTER VIII

Overcoming Challenges and Resistance

Addressing Skepticism and Misconceptions

It's critical to dispel myths and skepticism about herbal remedies for viral illnesses in order to promote knowledge, confidence, and well-informed choices among those looking for complementary or alternative methods of treating viral infections. With a long history that dates back thousands of years, herbal therapy provides a wide range of plant-based treatments that have been used historically to boost immune function, reduce symptoms, and enhance general wellness. Nevertheless, mistrust and misconceptions about herbal medicines continue despite an increasing amount of scientific evidence demonstrating their safety and usefulness. These are frequently caused by false information, cultural prejudices, and a lack of knowledge about the fundamentals and procedures of herbal therapy.

The idea that herbal remedies for viral infections are unsuccessful or subpar to traditional pharmaceutical therapies is a prevalent misunderstanding. Herbal medicines are dismissed by some critics as "folk medicine" or "alternative therapies," having no scientific backing for their efficacy or safety. Nonetheless, a plethora of research has evinced the antiviral characteristics of several herbs and botanical substances, underscoring their potential as adjunctive or substitute interventions for viral infections. Herbs that have been found to decrease viral replication, enhance immune function, and lessen the intensity as well as duration of symptoms associated with viral infections include echinacea, elderberry, licorice root, and astragalus. Practitioners can assist in debunking myths and fostering confidence in the efficacy and also safety of herbal treatments by informing people about the scientific evidence that supports their usage.

The idea that herbal remedies for viral problems are intrinsically dangerous or uncontrolled is another common misperception. Skeptics frequently raise issues with standardization, contamination, and quality control when claiming that herbal goods could be contaminated or contain dangerous ingredients that could endanger the public's health. While it is true that manufacturing processes and the nation of origin have a significant impact on the quality control and regulation of herbal products, many respectable herbal companies follow stringent quality standards and put their products through extensive testing to guarantee their safety, potency, and purity. Furthermore, customers need to be informed by herbalists and holistic health professionals about the safe and responsible use of herbal treatments, including dose guidelines, contraindications, and possible drug interactions. Practitioners might help address concerns regarding the security and dependability of herbal remedies for viral problems by fostering openness, responsibility, and customer understanding.

The idea that herbal remedies for viral problems are founded more on superstition, anecdotal evidence, or antiquated ideas than on scientific principles is a prevalent source of mistrust. Some critics discount herbal medicine as pseudoscientific or illogical, claiming that it is based on antiquated customs and cultural practices that have no place in contemporary culture. However, many herbal medicines undergo significant laboratory research, clinical trials, and systematic reviews to evaluate their efficacy, safety, and mechanism of action. This is because herbal therapy is based on rigorous scientific inquiry and empirical observation. In herbal medicine, empirical data and conventional wisdom are essential sources of information, but they shouldn't be the only factors used to assess the efficacy and safety of herbal treatments. Practitioners can help close the knowledge gap between traditional wisdom and contemporary science by having a conversation with skeptics about the scientific evidence supporting herbal medicine. This will assist in building a more nuanced and informed perspective on herbal remedies for viral problems.

Furthermore, institutional hurdles that restrict access to holistic healthcare options, socioeconomic inequities, and cultural biases can feed skepticism and misconceptions around herbal remedies for viral problems. Since traditional healing traditions have been marginalized by culture, historical injustices, and colonialism, herbal medicine is seen with distrust or mistrust in many cultures. People's opinions about herbal medicine and their capacity to get and pay for holistic healthcare treatments can also be influenced by socioeconomic factors, such as income, education, and accessibility to healthcare facilities. A multimodal strategy is needed to address these systemic problems, one that involves community-based education and outreach initiatives, healthcare personnel training in cultural competency, and lobbying for health equity. Practitioners can contribute to the development of a more equitable and accessible healthcare system that respects the various cultural viewpoints and healing traditions of all people by promoting inclusivity, diversity, and social justice in holistic healthcare.

In summary, clearing up doubts and disinformation about herbal remedies for viral illnesses is crucial to building confidence, understanding, and well-informed choices among those looking for complementary or alternative ways to treat viral infections. Practitioners can contribute to increasing trust in the use of herbal remedies for viral challenges and fostering a more inclusive as well as equitable healthcare system for all by educating people about the scientific evidence supporting the safety and also the efficacy of herbal remedies, encouraging transparency and accountability in the herbal industry, and conversing with skeptics about the institutional, socioeconomic, and cultural factors that shape perceptions of herbal medicine.

Navigating Legal and Regulatory Hurdles

When using herbal remedies for viral problems, practitioners and individuals must take into account the legal and regulatory obstacles that may arise. Herbal medicine is governed by a number of rules and regulations that control its production, sale, and use despite its long history of use and perceived therapeutic advantages. These national legal and regulatory systems present difficulties for consumers, holistic health professionals, and herbalists alike. It is crucial to comprehend and overcome these obstacles in order to maintain legal compliance, safeguard public health and safety, and advance accessibility to secure and reliable herbal treatments for viral infections.

A primary legal and regulatory consideration for herbal therapies for viral issues is whether they are classified as food products, dietary supplements, or pharmaceuticals. The intended use, therapeutic claims, and route of administration of herbal remedies determine whether they are regulated as dietary supplements or medications in numerous countries. To guarantee their safety, effectiveness, and quality, medicines must meet strict regulatory requirements, such as pre-market approval, clinical studies, and quality control standards. Conversely, dietary supplements are often covered by rules pertaining to food products and are less strictly regulated. In order to guarantee adherence to relevant rules and regulations and steer clear of legal problems, practitioners and customers alike must comprehend the regulatory classification of herbal products.

The problem of product labeling, marketing, and advertising presents another legal and regulatory barrier for herbal remedies for viral problems. Herbal products must have accurate and truthful labeling that includes information about the product's ingredients, dosage, usage instructions, possible adverse effects, and contraindications. This requirement applies to many nations. Furthermore, it is frequently forbidden for herbal medicines to make any unsupported medicinal or health claims that are not backed up by scientific data. Manufacturers, distributors, and retailers risk legal action, fines, or penalties for breaking labeling and advertising requirements. Both consumers and practitioners need to be aware of these rules and make sure they only buy and recommend herbal items from reliable vendors who abide by the law.

Another essential factor to take into account when choosing herbal remedies for viral problems is quality control and production standards. Regulations governing the cultivation, manufacturing, and distribution of herbal products are in place to guarantee their quality, safety, and purity. These guidelines cover the sourcing of raw materials, manufacturing processes, packaging, labeling, and storage. Herbal goods are kept free of pollutants, adulterants, and other impurities that could endanger public health when Good Manufacturing Practices (GMP) rules are followed. It is recommended that consumers and practitioners look for herbal products made by companies that follow GMP guidelines and submit them to independent testing in order to ensure their quality and purity.

Furthermore, depending on the particular herbs and botanical elements employed in their composition, herbal remedies for viral problems can be subject to additional rules and limits. Certain herbs are governed by international treaties that control their usage, commerce, harvesting, and production, or they are categorized as controlled substances. For example, because of their potential for abuse, dependence, or adverse health impacts, plants like ephedra, kratom, and cannabis are governed by stringent restrictions. Furthermore, some herbs have the potential to mix with pharmaceuticals or be contraindicated for people with particular medical conditions, so healthcare experts must carefully examine and supervise their use. When employing herbal remedies for viral problems, practitioners and consumers should be aware of these rules and limitations and seek advice from licensed herbalists or healthcare specialists.

In conclusion, using herbal remedies for viral problems involves a complex but necessary process of managing legal and regulatory obstacles. Critical factors for practitioners and consumers to take into account include knowing the classification of herbal products, adhering to labeling and advertising regulations, maintaining quality control and manufacturing standards, and being aware of additional regulations and restrictions for particular herbs. Stakeholders can cooperate to get past legal and regulatory obstacles and advance access to safe and efficient herbal remedies for viral challenges by remaining informed about relevant laws and regulations, advocating for fair and equitable access to herbal remedies, and encouraging transparency and accountability in the herbal industry.

Overcoming Cultural and Societal Barriers

Herbal remedies for viral problems must be widely accepted and adopted in order to overcome social and cultural barriers. Social conventions, institutional structures, and cultural views can all have an impact on people's attitudes about herbal medicine and their openness to trying out complementary or alternative methods of treating viral infections. Herbal medicine practitioners and advocates can contribute to creating a more welcoming and also inclusive atmosphere for herbal medicine as a feasible solution for viral issues by addressing these obstacles and advancing awareness, education, and inclusivity.

A major cultural obstacle to the use of herbal remedies for viral infections is the belief that herbal treatment is a kind of traditional or folk medicine with no scientific backing or legitimacy. Herbal medicines have been a part of traditional healing techniques for ages in many cultures. These traditions have been passed down through the generations based on experiential wisdom and empirical understanding. However, compared to traditional pharmaceutical therapies, which are seen as more scientific and evidence-based, herbal medicine is frequently seen as antiquated or primitive in modern society. It will take education and awareness-raising initiatives to present the scientific evidence for the safety and effectiveness of herbal medicines for viral infections in order to overcome this cultural bias. Practitioners and advocates can contribute to bridging the knowledge gap between traditional wisdom and contemporary scientific understanding by promoting evidence-based herbal medicine and debunking myths and misconceptions. This will increase acceptance and confidence in herbal remedies for viral problems.

Social hurdles that affect people's access to and use of herbal medicine for viral problems include socioeconomic inequality, healthcare access, and cultural competence. Access to holistic health choices, such as herbal medicine, is sometimes restricted in many communities by socioeconomic status, educational attainment, place of residence, and cultural background. Furthermore, people's views of health and sickness can be influenced by cultural customs and beliefs, which can also affect their preferences for healthcare providers and treatment approaches. A multimodal strategy is needed to overcome these obstacles, one that involves expanding access to holistic health services, supporting social justice and health equity, and encouraging cultural competency and sensitivity among healthcare professionals. In order to ensure that everyone has equitable access to herbal medicines for viral infections, practitioners and advocates should work to eliminate barriers to access and promote diversity and inclusivity in alternative medicine.

Moreover, institutional impediments, including insurance coverage, healthcare policies, and regulatory restrictions, might make it more challenging to incorporate herbal therapy into traditional healthcare systems. Restrictions governing the manufacturing, sale, and use of herbal remedies are applicable in many countries. These restrictions may differ significantly based on the jurisdiction and regulatory structure. Furthermore, insurance and healthcare policies do not always cover or support holistic health services, such as consultations and treatments using herbal medicine. Advocacy and policy reform are needed to break down these institutional barriers in order to support the integration of herbal medicine into traditional healthcare systems, expand insurance coverage for holistic health services, and guarantee that laws are just, equitable, and supportive of the safe and efficient use of herbal remedies for viral infections. Practitioners and activists can contribute to the development of an atmosphere that encourages the incorporation of herbal medicine into conventional healthcare systems and facilitates everyone's access to holistic health solutions by pushing for legislative and regulatory reform.

In conclusion, societal and cultural barriers must be removed in order for herbal remedies for viral problems to be widely accepted and used. Herbal medicine can effectively treat viral infections in a more welcoming and inclusive environment if cultural biases, socioeconomic disparities, healthcare access, cultural competence, institutional limitations, and regulatory barriers are addressed. Practitioners and advocates can also play a significant role in fostering this environment. Stakeholders can collaborate to remove obstacles to care, advance diversity and equity in holistic health care, and guarantee that everyone has equitable access to safe and efficient herbal remedies for viral infections through lobbying, education, and policy reform.

Future Directions and Opportunities

With increased interest and study in the realm of botanical medicine, there are promising future avenues and opportunities for herbal treatments in addressing viral issues. In order to prevent and treat viral infections, there is a growing focus on investigating natural alternatives, such as herbal medicines, as the globe struggles with new viral threats and rising antibiotic resistance. Novel strategies for utilizing plants' medicinal potential to treat viral infections are becoming possible thanks to developments in science, technology, and integrative medicine.

Finding and creating new antiviral components from medicinal plants is one of the main areas in which herbal remedies for viral problems can be used in the future. Through developments in high-throughput screening methods, phytochemistry, and bioinformatics, scientists are finding bioactive substances in plants that have strong antiviral properties against a variety of viruses. These substances, which may have less adverse effects and a decreased chance of resistance development than traditional antiviral medications, include flavonoids, alkaloids, polyphenols, and terpenoids. Scientists are finding new directions for the creation of herbal remedies and botanical supplements for viral infections by utilizing the power of nature's pharmacy.

Herbal therapies for viral issues could also take the route of fusing traditional knowledge with state-of-the-art scientific approaches to optimize therapeutic efficacy and safety. Herbal treatments have long been used in traditional medical systems, including Ayurveda, Traditional Chinese Medicine (TCM), and Indigenous healing practices, to treat viral infections and strengthen the immune system. Practitioners and researchers can find synergistic herbal combinations, dosage forms, and delivery systems that improve the bioavailability and therapeutic effects of herbal treatments by fusing traditional wisdom with evidence-based research. Furthermore, scientists may verify the safety and effectiveness of conventional herbal preparations for viral problems through observational studies and clinical trials, giving traditional therapeutic methods much-needed legitimacy and validity.

Furthermore, personalized medicine approaches that customize treatment plans to individual genetic, environmental, and lifestyle factors hold promise for future herbal remedies for viral infections. The fields of systems biology, metabolomics, and genomic medicine have advanced, providing researchers with a new understanding of the molecular mechanisms behind viral infections and host-pathogen interactions. Through an awareness of the ways in which genetic differences and environmental circumstances affect a person's susceptibility to viral infections and how the body responds to treatment, herbal practitioners can create customized protocols that maximize benefits and reduce side effects. Personalized medicine methods allow individuals to take an active role in their health care, which encourages a more patient-centered and all-encompassing approach to viral problems.

Future research on herbal remedies for viral problems may also look into synergistic therapies, which integrate herbal remedies with other approaches like diet, lifestyle modifications, and mind-body techniques. The utilization of holistic techniques that target the root causes of viral infections and foster general health and well-being may improve treatment results and lower the likelihood of recurrence. Practitioners can offer complete and integrative care that addresses the mental, emotional, and physical elements of viral problems by combining herbal medicine with complementary therapies. This multifaceted approach to healing provides new opportunities to investigate the synergy between herbal treatments and other therapeutic techniques and is in line with integrative medicine tenets.

In conclusion, with increased interest and study in the field of botanical medicine, future paths and potential for herbal remedies for viral issues seem promising. Practitioners and researchers can advance the development and use of herbal remedies for managing viral infections by embracing personalized medicine approaches, embracing the power of nature's pharmacy, exploring synergistic therapies, and fusing traditional wisdom with cutting-edge scientific methods. Herbal medicine has the potential to significantly contribute to reducing the worldwide burden of viral diseases and enhancing health and well-being for people and communities everywhere with sustained investment in research, education, and innovation.

CHAPTER IX

Herbal Remedies in Traditional Medicine Systems

Ayurveda and Herbal Antiviral Practices

For thousands of years, herbal medicines have been an essential component of Ayurvedic therapy, providing a comprehensive strategy for mental, physical, and spiritual well-being. Herbs are revered as holy gifts from nature in Ayurveda, the age-old Indian medical system, and are utilized to prevent and cure a variety of illnesses, including viral infections. In order to restore harmony and balance to the body's doshas or constitutional types, Ayurvedic herbs are chosen and prepared according to their energetics, tastes, and therapeutic capabilities. Practitioners can harness the healing power of nature to improve immune function, reduce symptoms, and promote overall well-being by combining Ayurvedic herbal remedies with antiviral therapies.

The idea of dinacharya, or daily routine, is central to Ayurveda and highlights the need to uphold healthy habits and lifestyle practices in order to prevent disease and encourage longevity. Dinacharya heavily relies on Ayurvedic herbal medicines, which include the use of turmeric, ginger, and tulsi (holy basil) to boost immunity, improve digestion, and encourage vigor. These herbs are frequently utilized to nourish the body and ward against imbalances that can result in viral illnesses. Examples of these rituals include adding them to morning tea or spice-infused meals. People can strengthen their body's natural defense mechanisms and lower their risk of viral diseases by incorporating Ayurvedic herbs into their everyday routines.

Ayurvedic herbs not only promote general health and well-being but also specifically target viral infections and the symptoms that accompany them. Strong antiviral qualities found in many Ayurvedic medicines help prevent viral replication, strengthen the immune system, and reduce symptoms like fever, coughing, and exhaustion. For instance, neem, a bitter and calming herb, is well known for its immune-stimulating, antiviral, and antibacterial qualities, which make it a valuable treatment for viral illnesses like herpes, the flu, and colds. Likewise, during periods of elevated stress or immune suppression, ashwagandha, an adaptogenic herb, helps the body adjust to stress and maintains immunological function, which makes it helpful for managing and avoiding viral infections. People can strengthen their body's defenses against viral threats and expedite their recuperation from disease by combining these and other Ayurvedic medicines into antiviral treatments.

Rasayanas, sometimes called chyawanprash, are Ayurvedic herbal compositions intended to boost immunity and extend life. Herbs, spices, and other natural ingredients are carefully chosen and blended into these formulas to maximize their synergistic benefits and therapeutic potency. For instance, amla (Indian gooseberry), ashwagandha, and guduchi are some of the herbs used to make the traditional Ayurvedic tonic known as chyawanprash. Other ingredients include honey, ghee, and other nutritious elements. Because of its ability to boost immunity, chyawanprash is frequently used to treat and also prevent respiratory illnesses and wildly viral infections. People can boost their immunity and become more resistant to viral infections by adding Ayurvedic herbal formulations into their daily routine.

Moreover, to enhance general health and well-being, Ayurvedic herbal medicines are frequently combined with other Ayurvedic therapies, including pranayama (breathing exercises), yoga, meditation, and panchakarma (detoxification). For instance, panchakarma is a revitalizing and cleansing therapy that uses a range of detoxification procedures, such as massage, herbal steam baths, and enemas, to flush out toxins from the body and balance the doshas. People who have collected toxins and impurities might strengthen their immune systems and become more vulnerable to viral infections by undergoing panchakarma therapy. Similar to this, Ayurvedic herbal therapies for antiviral techniques benefit significantly from the addition of yoga, meditation, and pranayama as they aid in stress reduction, relaxation, and immune system enhancement.

To sum up, Ayurvedic herbal treatments combine age-old knowledge with cutting-edge scientific research to provide a comprehensive strategy for treating viral infections that enhances health and well-being across the board. People can assist their body's natural defensive systems and encourage a quicker recovery from disease by incorporating Ayurvedic herbs into their daily routines, employing Ayurvedic formulations and therapies to improve the immune system, and using particular herbal remedies to target viral infections. Herbal antiviral treatments can be enhanced and complemented by Ayurveda, which emphasizes balance, harmony, and personalized care. This holistic approach offers a comprehensive way to manage viral issues and promote optimal health and wellness.

Traditional Chinese Medicine (TCM) Approaches

Herbal medicines have long been an integral part of Traditional Chinese Medicine's (TCM) holistic approach to health and wellness. Traditional Chinese Medicine (TCM), whose roots date back thousands of years, views the human body as a complex system of meridians, or related energy channels, that transmit qi, or life force, through them. According to TCM theory, diseases and illnesses, including viral infections, can result from imbalances or blockages in the movement of qi. Herbal medicine is essential for addressing the underlying causes of sickness, promoting general well-being, and reestablishing harmony as well as balance in the body's energy system.

The idea of yin and yang, which stand for the dualistic forces of nature that are constantly changing and in balance, is one of the fundamental ideas of TCM. According to TCM belief, disease results from imbalances or interruptions in the body's harmonic balance between yin and yang. Health is attained when this equilibrium is maintained. In TCM, herbal treatments are used to balance the yin and yang energies, tonify deficiencies, eliminate excesses, and improve the body's defenses against viral diseases. For instance, warming herbs like ginger and cinnamon are used to drive away cold and fortify the body's defenses against external infections. In contrast, cooling herbs like mint and chrysanthemum are used to eliminate excess heat and inflammation associated with viral fevers.

Additionally, TCM uses an advanced system of classifying herbs according to their energy qualities, flavor profiles, and medicinal effects. Herbalists can choose herbs that target individual patterns of disharmony and symptoms by classifying them based on their temperature (cooling, warming, or neutral), flavor (sour, bitter, sweet, pungent, or salty), and therapeutic actions (tonifying, dispersing, draining, etc.). Herbs that are categorized as tonifying, including ginseng and astragalus, enhance the body's qi and immune system, making them effective treatments for both curing and preventing viral infections. Similarly, herbs that are good for treating viral fevers and inflammatory disorders include forsythia and honeysuckle, which are categorized as dispersing herbs that remove heat and toxins from the body.

Many TCM herbs have strong antiviral qualities in addition to their therapeutic benefits, which support immune system development, prevent viral replication, and lessen the symptoms of viral illnesses. Herbs with proven anti-replication properties, such as licorice root and Isatis leaf, include bioactive components that prevent the growth of influenza viruses and other respiratory diseases. Similar to this, recent research supports the traditional usage of plants like honeysuckle and forsythia, which have antiviral action against a broad spectrum of pathogens, to treat viral diseases like the flu and the common cold. TCM practitioners can offer thorough and efficient therapy for viral infections by combining these and other antiviral herbs into herbal formulae. This allows them to address both the underlying causes of illness and the symptoms linked to viral disorders.

TCM also stresses the significance of customized care based on each person's distinct constitution, pattern of disharmony, and symptoms. Traditional Chinese medicine practitioners identify underlying imbalances or vulnerabilities that may predispose a patient to viral infections by a thorough assessment of the patient's medical history, lifestyle choices, and tongue and pulse diagnosis. Using the results of this evaluation, practitioners can customize herbal remedies to target and individually treat viral problems by addressing the unique patterns of disharmony and symptoms that each patient presents with. A greater comprehension and appreciation of the holistic principles of Traditional Chinese Medicine (TCM) are fostered by this tailored approach to care, which also improves treatment outcomes and gives patients the power to participate actively in their health management.

Additionally, TCM herbal treatment frequently makes use of intricate concoctions called herbal formulas or prescriptions, which are made up of several carefully chosen herbs that are mixed to maximize their medicinal potency and synergistic effects. Rather than only treating symptoms, these formulae aim to address the complex nature of sickness and address its underlying causes. For instance, the traditional TCM prescription yin qiao san uses a combination of herbs, including gypsum, honeysuckle, and forsythia, to resolve toxins, clear heat, and relieve fever, sore throat, and headache symptoms caused by viral infections. Similar to this, gui zhi tang is a beneficial remedy for treating colds and flu that cause chills and body aches. It mixes cinnamon twig, peony root, and licorice root to dissipate cold, warm the interior, and increase perspiration. TCM practitioners can provide targeted and successful therapy for viral problems by utilizing herbal formulae that address the unique patterns of disharmony and symptoms that each patient presents with. This supports the body's intrinsic healing power and promotes optimal health and well-being.

In summary, herbal medicines are essential to Traditional Chinese Medicine's (TCM) management of viral infections because they provide a customized, all-encompassing approach to health and well-being. Because TCM herbal medicine addresses the underlying causes of illness, promotes general well-being, and restores harmony and balance to the body's energy system, it provides a comprehensive and effective treatment alternative for viral infections. Herbal medicine (TCM) offers valuable insights and practices that complement and enhance herbal antiviral approaches, offering a holistic and integrative approach to managing viral infections and promoting optimal health and wellness. TCM places an emphasis on yin and yang balance, herbal classification, individualized treatment, and complex herbal formulations.

Indigenous Herbal Healing Practices

Indigenous healing techniques have included herbal treatments for millennia as a reflection of their profound connection to the land, plants, and natural world. Indigenous communities all around the world have created complex herbal medicine systems based on traditional knowledge that has been handed down through the years by elders, shamans, and healers. These herbal remedies emphasize a holistic approach to health as well as wellness that takes into account all facets of existence—physical, mental, emotional, and spiritual— and are firmly anchored in the spiritual, cultural, and ecological traditions of Indigenous peoples.

Indigenous herbal healing traditions are based on the understanding that all living things are interrelated and that it is crucial to preserve harmony and balance with the natural environment. Native American healers are aware that plants are holy gifts from the Earth with great healing potential that should be treated with appreciation, respect, and care. Indigenous peoples have gained profound insights into the medicinal characteristics of indigenous plants and how to use them to heal a wide range of diseases, including viral infections, by developing a reciprocal relationship with the land and its inhabitants.

The belief in the innate knowledge and intelligence of nature is reflected in the use of plants in their complete, unprocessed form in Indigenous herbal healing methods. Gathering plants from their native environments while paying close attention to moon phases, seasonal cycles, and ceremonial rituals, indigenous healers honor the plant's spirit and give prayers of thanks for its therapeutic properties. With utmost regard for the fragile balance of ecosystems and the interdependent web of life, plants are collected in an ethical and also sustainable manner. Indigenous healers preserve the health and quantity of medicinal plants for future generations by carefully harvesting them in compliance with customary practices.

Indigenous herbal healing approaches also place a strong emphasis on the value of intergenerational knowledge transfer and cultural continuity, with elders teaching younger generations traditional healing techniques through storytelling, oral tradition, and practical apprenticeship. The lived experiences, observations, and insights of Indigenous peoples, who have developed close relationships with the land and its inhabitants over millennia, serve as the foundation for this knowledge transfer. Indigenous communities regain their sovereignty, resilience, and self-determination in the face of historical traumas, colonial oppression, and environmental destruction by protecting and reviving traditional healing techniques.

Moreover, Indigenous herbal healing methods are intricately linked to ceremonial and spiritual traditions, illustrating a holistic view of health and wellness that takes into account all aspects of existence—mental, emotional, spiritual, and physical. In addition to being used as sources of physical medicine, plants are also seen as allies, instructors, and guides for people seeking healing and wholeness. Sweat lodges, plant medicine ceremonies, and smudging are among the revered and intentional traditions that call upon the knowledge and healing power of the natural world to help individuals and communities find harmony and balance again.

Indigenous herbal treatments are prized for their solid therapeutic qualities and capacity to treat a variety of illnesses, including viral infections, in addition to their spiritual and ceremonial significance. Antiviral solid, immune-stimulating, and anti-inflammatory qualities found in many indigenous plants aid in bolstering the body's natural defenses and advancing healing. For instance, Indigenous peoples have traditionally used herbs like osha root, elderberry, and echinacea to cure and prevent respiratory diseases, including pneumonia, the flu, and colds. These plants are essential partners in the fight against viral infections because they contain bioactive chemicals that support immune function, reduce inflammation, and limit viral reproduction.

Additionally, traditional techniques, including decoction, infusion, tincture, and poultice, are frequently used to produce indigenous herbal treatments, aiding in the extraction and preservation of the plant's therapeutic qualities. These medications are applied topically, orally, or by inhalation, according to the individual's needs and symptoms. Indigenous healers tailor their therapies to address the root causes of sickness and reestablish bodily, mental, and spiritual balance by drawing on their vast understanding of plant energetics, tastes, and therapeutic actions.

To sum up, indigenous herbal treatment methods, which are based on traditional knowledge, cultural continuity, and spiritual understanding, provide a thorough and all-encompassing approach to treating viral infections. Indigenous peoples have gained significant insights into the therapeutic qualities of native plants and their uses for enhancing health and wellness by respecting the interdependence of all living things and the holiness of the natural world. Indigenous communities are recovering and reviving their traditional healing practices through cultural revitalization efforts, community-led initiatives, and cooperative partnerships. These communities are providing insightful analysis and practical solutions for dealing with viral challenges and advancing holistic health and well-being for everybody.

Integrating Global Herbal Traditions

For thousands of years, herbal remedies have been an essential component of healing customs in many cultures and regions, demonstrating a solid bond with the land, plants, and natural world. Herbal therapy has been essential to supporting health and wellness on all levels of being, from the traditional African, Native American, and other indigenous healing techniques to the age-old Ayurvedic and Traditional Chinese therapy (TCM) systems. As the world becomes increasingly interconnected and diversified, there is a growing recognition of the significance of integrating global herbal traditions to address the complex health concerns that contemporary humanity faces.

Acknowledging the diversity of healing practices and the universality of healing principles is one of the fundamental tenets of the integration of herbal traditions worldwide. There are similar themes and beliefs that unify herbal traditions, such as the value of holistic health, the connectivity of mind, body, and spirit, and the healing power of nature, even though each tradition has its own distinct methods, philosophies, and cultural contexts. By appreciating and respecting the diversity of herbal traditions, professionals can draw from a vast reservoir of knowledge and understanding to create complete and successful treatment programs that are customized to the particular requirements and circumstances of each patient.

The incorporation of diverse herbal traditions also provides insightful viewpoints that can improve and enrich the practice of herbal therapy. Every herbal tradition offers a different set of botanical resources, treatment modalities, diagnostic techniques, and therapeutic philosophies, resulting in a comprehensive and complex approach to healing. Ayurveda, for instance, places great emphasis on constitutional types and customized care, whereas TCM uses herbal medicine, acupuncture, and other techniques to balance the body's energy system. By combining these many methods, professionals can create individualized treatment programs that target the underlying causes of disease and advance each patient's best possible state of health and wellness.

Furthermore, the blending of various herbal traditions from throughout the world promotes intercultural communication, cooperation, and respect between healers and practitioners from various traditions and backgrounds. Practitioners can expand their awareness of herbal medicine as a universal healing modality, learn from one another, and broaden their perspectives by exchanging best practices, knowledge, and experiences. Innovative approaches to addressing health difficulties, such as viral infections, chronic diseases, and mental health disorders, can result from collaborative relationships involving traditional healers, herbalists, academics, and healthcare providers. Together, practitioners can build comprehensive, culturally aware solutions that benefit people and communities by utilizing the advantages of each tradition.

Furthermore, the incorporation of worldwide herbal customs encourages conservation, sustainability, and ethical procurement of therapeutic plants. A lot of conventional herbal treatments use plants that have been farmed or wildcrafted and collected according to customs and procedures. Herbalists can contribute to the preservation of biodiversity, the protection of endangered plant species, and also the support of local communities that depend on medicinal herbs for their livelihoods by incorporating ethical and sustainable harvesting practices into their work. In addition, by encouraging the growing of medicinal plants in farms, gardens, and public areas, practitioners can guarantee a long-term supply of premium herbs for the coming generations.

In addition, the amalgamation of worldwide herbal customs provides significant perspectives and remedies for managing the intricate health issues confronting humanity presently, including viral infections, antibiotic resistance, persistent illnesses, and psychological problems. A comprehensive as well as integrated approach to health and well-being that prioritizes empowerment, balance, and prevention is offered by herbal medicine. The integration of herbal remedies into healthcare systems, along with the promotion of public education and awareness and interdisciplinary collaboration, can facilitate the integration of complementary and conventional medicine, increase accessibility to holistic healthcare, and advance global health and well-being for individuals and communities.

Conclusively, the amalgamation of worldwide herbal customs presents a potent and revolutionary method of therapy that respects the diversity of cultures, viewpoints, and therapeutic techniques. By respecting and embracing the wisdom of traditional healing systems, practitioners can leverage a wealth of knowledge and also experience to develop comprehensive and effective treatment programs that address the underlying causes of illness and promote everyone's optimal health and wellness. Practitioners may collaborate to find creative answers to the complex health issues that humanity faces today through cross-cultural interaction, respect, and cooperation. This will result in a more inclusive, long-lasting, and comprehensive approach to healthcare that will benefit future generations.

CHAPTER X

Herbal Medicine and Public Health

Role of Herbal Medicine in Pandemic Preparedness

Recent years have seen a significant increase in interest in the role of herbal medicine in pandemic preparedness, especially in light of the COVID-19 pandemic that is still running strong and the need for efficient methods to control, prevent, and lessen the transmission of infectious diseases. With a lengthy history of use in conventional medical systems all over the world, herbal medicine provides insightful information and practical recommendations for pandemic preparedness, including supportive care, treatment, and prevention. Herbal medicine has the potential to significantly improve resilience and fortify public health systems in the face of pandemics by utilizing the therapeutic potential of medicinal plants, fusing traditional knowledge with contemporary science, and promoting sustainable and culturally sensitive healthcare practices.

The focus herbal medicine places on immune support and prevention makes it one of the main assets to pandemic preparedness. Firm immune-stimulating, anti-inflammatory, and antiviral qualities found in many medicinal plants support the body's natural defenses against illness and lower its risk of infection. Traditional medical systems have long employed herbs like echinacea, elderberry, and astragalus to strengthen the immune system, increase resistance to illnesses, and enhance general health and vitality. Through daily routines that incorporate these and other immune-supporting herbs, people can strengthen their immune systems, lessen their vulnerability to viral illnesses, and slow down the spread of pandemics.

Moreover, a multitude of botanical resources are available in herbal therapy to cure viral infections and the symptoms that accompany them. Bioactive substances found in a variety of medicinal plants have been demonstrated to prevent the spread of viruses, lessen inflammation, ease respiratory symptoms, and aid in the healing process. Herbs that have shown antiviral efficacy against a variety of respiratory viruses, including influenza and coronaviruses, include licorice root, Isatis leaf, and honeysuckle. Herbalists may effectively and supportively care for patients impacted by pandemics by creating herbal treatments that specifically target the mechanisms of viral pathogenesis. This can assist to lessen the severity and duration of sickness and enhance clinical results.

Herbal medicine also provides practical ways to treat the adverse effects of pandemics on mental and emotional health, such as stress, anxiety, depression, and social isolation. Numerous therapeutic herbs have nervine, adaptogenic, and anxiolytic qualities that aid in stress reduction, relaxation, and emotional resilience. Herbs that have long been used to ease anxiety, elevate mood, and enhance sleep quality include chamomile, holy basil, and ashwagandha. Practitioners can support mental health, build resilience and coping mechanisms, and assist patients in managing the psychological effects of pandemics by combining these and other herbal treatments into comprehensive therapy plans.

Herbal medicine also provides a culturally aware and sustainable approach to healthcare that honors indigenous peoples' customs and the planet's ecological integrity. The viability and availability of medicinal plants for future generations are ensured by employing sustainable methods and protocols to harvest plants, either wildcrafted or farmed, for many traditional herbal treatments. Practitioners can contribute to the preservation of traditional knowledge, biodiversity protection, and the assistance of indigenous populations that rely on medicinal plants for their livelihoods by encouraging the ethical sourcing, conservation, and care of medicinal plants.

Furthermore, tackling the systemic injustices and socioeconomic gaps that worsen the effects of pandemics on vulnerable groups is something that herbal therapy may help with. Herbal treatments are a financially viable and inclusive healthcare option for areas with limited access to traditional medical services since many medicinal plants are widely available, reasonably priced, and accessible to people of all income levels. Herbal medicine has the potential to close the gap between conventional and complementary medicine, increase access to holistic healthcare, advance social justice and health equity, and empower local healers and herbalists through the promotion of community-based healthcare initiatives and partnerships with healthcare providers.

Herbal medicine also provides chances for multidisciplinary study and collaboration to advance our knowledge of the therapeutic potential of medicinal plants and how to use them for pandemic preparedness.

Researchers can confirm the effectiveness, safety, and mechanisms of action of herbal treatments for treating and preventing viral infections by carrying out meticulous scientific investigations, clinical trials, and observational studies. Practitioners and researchers can create evidence-based recommendations, protocols, and best practices for integrating herbal medicine into public health strategies and pandemic preparation plans by fusing traditional knowledge with contemporary scientific approaches.

In summary, herbal medicine has a broad and diverse role in pandemic preparedness, including treatment, prevention, mental health, sustainability, cultural sensitivity, health equity, and scientific research. Herbal medicine has the potential to improve resilience significantly, fortify public health systems, and lessen the effects of pandemics on people and communities all over the world by utilizing the therapeutic potential of medicinal plants, to fuse traditional knowledge with contemporary science, and to encourage holistic and inclusive approaches to healthcare. Herbal medicine can significantly improve pandemic preparedness and the security of global health for future generations if research, education, and community empowerment are sustained.

Community-Based Herbal Healthcare Initiatives

Using ancient healing methods, medicinal plants, and holistic healthcare techniques, community-based herbal healthcare projects offer a grassroots approach to health and well-being that enables people and communities to take charge of their own health. These programs, which seek to meet the healthcare requirements of underprivileged and marginalized people, advance health equity, and bolster community resilience, are based on the values of self-reliance, sustainability, cultural continuity, and social justice. Community-based herbal healthcare projects promote prevention, empowerment, and holistic well-being through empowering local healers, herbalists, healthcare providers, and community members to form relationships. This collaborative and participatory approach to healthcare is essential.

An essential tenet of community-based herbal healthcare programs is the appreciation of the role that local customs, knowledge, and resources play in fostering health and well-being. Herbal medicine and traditional healing techniques are part of a rich legacy of many cultures worldwide, handed down through the decades by shamans, elders, and healers. Communities can access an invaluable reservoir of knowledge and wisdom anchored in the land, culture, and lived experiences of the people by recovering and reviving these ancestral healing practices. The identification, harvesting, preparation, and use of medicinal plants for the promotion of health and treatment of common ailments can be taught to individuals through community-led efforts to preserve and disseminate traditional knowledge.

Initiatives for community-based herbal healthcare also highlight the value of integrative and holistic approaches to well-being that take into account the connection between the mind, body, and spirit. Ayurveda, Traditional Chinese Medicine (TCM), and indigenous healing methods are just a few examples of traditional healing systems that emphasize treating the whole person as opposed to only the disease's symptoms. Community-based healthcare initiatives integrate herbal remedies, dietary and lifestyle interventions, mind-body practices, and social support networks to provide a personalized and all-encompassing approach to disease prevention and health promotion. This approach enables individuals to participate actively in their own healing process.

Furthermore, by addressing the underlying social, economic, and environmental determinants of health that contribute to health disparities and inequities, community-based herbal healthcare efforts advance social justice and health equity. Conventional medical care is not readily available to many underprivileged and oppressed populations because of things like racism, poverty, remote location, and cultural barriers.

Community-based herbal efforts can help close the gap between conventional and complementary medicine, increase access to holistic healthcare, and advance health equity for all by offering inexpensive, easily accessible, and culturally relevant healthcare services. Additionally, these programs can assist communities in developing self-reliance, resilience, and solidarity by enabling individuals and groups to actively participate in their own health care, which can generate a sense of collective agency and empowerment.

In addition, by encouraging the sustainable cultivation, wildcrafting, and conservation of medicinal plants, community-based herbal healthcare projects support ecological stewardship and environmental sustainability. The utilization of wildcrafted or cultivated plants that are obtained with sustainable methods and protocols is a crucial component of many traditional healing practices. This ensures that medicinal plants will remain abundant and necessary for future generations. Community-based herbal projects can contribute to biodiversity conservation, traditional knowledge preservation, and the uplift of local economies that depend on medicinal plants for their livelihoods. They do this by encouraging ethical sourcing, conservation, and management of medicinal plants. Furthermore, these projects can contribute to the development of a greater understanding and respect for the interconnection of all life and the significance of living in harmony with the Earth by reestablishing a connection between individual communities and the natural environment.

Furthermore, by offering instruction, workshops, and resources on herbal medicine, nutrition, gardening, and holistic health practices, community-based herbal healthcare projects support empowerment, education, and the development of self-care skills. By providing people with the necessary information, abilities, and resources to manage their own health and wellness, these programs can enable communities to become more resilient, self-sufficient, and proactive in their health care.

Community-based herbal projects can also contribute to the development of social capital and the strengthening of social networks within communities by promoting a culture of solidarity, mutual support, and collective action. This can create a sense of connection, belonging, and shared purpose.

In conclusion, via the use of medicinal plants, conventional treatment methods, and holistic healthcare modalities, community-based herbal healthcare programs offer a grassroots approach to health and well-being that enables people and communities to take charge of their own health. These programs provide a revolutionary approach to healthcare that targets the root causes of disease and advances everyone's health and well-being by reclaiming and reviving traditional healing practices, supporting environmental sustainability, advancing social justice and health equity, and promoting knowledge, self- care abilities, and empowerment. Community-based herbal healthcare programs have the potential to significantly contribute to the development of healthier, more resilient, and more equitable communities for future generations, provided they receive sustained support and funding.

Herbal Medicine in Resource-limited Settings

In resource-constrained environments where access to traditional healthcare is either restricted or nonexistent, herbal medicine is essential. In these situations, medicinal plants play a crucial role in healthcare provision by offering readily available, reasonably priced, and culturally appropriate solutions to address community healthcare requirements. Resource-limited settings include a broad spectrum of locations, such as isolated and rural regions, low-income urban neighborhoods, camps for refugees, and indigenous communities. These settings are characterized by socioeconomic inequality, political unrest, geographic isolation, and environmental difficulties, all of which limit access to healthcare services. Herbal medicine, which recognizes the interdependence of people and their surroundings, provides a comprehensive and integrative approach to health and wellness in such circumstances. This approach addresses the mental, emotional, physical, and spiritual aspects of well-being.

Herbal medicine has several benefits, two of which are its cost and accessibility in environments with low resources. Numerous therapeutic plants can be found easily in the surrounding area, either growing wild or being grown in fields, forests, and home gardens. Herbal remedies are frequently available to people of all income levels, in contrast to traditional drugs, which can be costly and also challenging to obtain. This makes them a viable and affordable healthcare choice for populations with low financial resources. Furthermore, by giving people the information, abilities, and tools necessary to cultivate, harvest, prepare, and utilize medicinal plants for promoting health and treating common disorders, herbal medicine empowers people to take charge of their own health.

Additionally, in situations with limited resources, herbal therapy provides community-centered, culturally appropriate answers to healthcare problems. A solid connection to the earth, ancestors, and spiritual worlds is reflected in the many traditional healing techniques that have their roots in the cultural traditions, beliefs, and values of indigenous peoples and local communities. By integrating traditional healing methods into healthcare systems, professionals can promote a sense of pride, identity, and self-determination among communities by honoring and respecting the cultural legacy and wisdom of the people. Herbal medicine can also support intergenerational solidarity, social cohesion, and the revitalization of cultural traditions by enlisting community members in the transmission and preservation of traditional knowledge.

Herbal medicine also provides integrative and holistic methods to wellness that target the underlying causes of disease and enhance general health. Numerous medicinal plants have complex medicinal qualities that affect the immunological, neurological, digestive, and cardiovascular systems, among other bodily systems. In resource-constrained contexts, practitioners can address the complex interaction of physical, mental, emotional, and environmental aspects that contribute to disease burden and health inequities by adding herbal treatments into holistic treatment plans. Herbal medicine also places a strong emphasis on lifestyle changes, preventative measures, and self-care routines that enable people to take charge of their health and delay the emergence of chronic illnesses.

Herbal therapy also provides ecologically benign and long-lasting answers to medical problems in resource-constrained environments. Unlike conventional pharmaceuticals, which may have adverse environmental effects due to chemical pollution, deforestation, and overharvesting of wild species, herbal remedies are made from renewable and biodegradable plant sources that can be grown, harvested, and processed sustainably. Advocates for ethical sourcing, conservation, and care of medicinal plants can contribute to the preservation of ecosystems, biodiversity, and local economies that rely on medicinal plants for their subsistence. Herbal medicine can also promote a greater understanding and respect for the interdependence of all life and the significance of living in balance with the environment by reestablishing a connection between individuals and communities and the natural world.

Additionally, in environments with limited resources, herbal medicine presents chances for capacity building, self-reliance, and community empowerment. Oral tradition, storytelling, and practical apprenticeship are among the ways that many traditional healing techniques are passed down, allowing information and abilities to be passed down within families and communities from one generation to the next. Through the provision of herbal medicine education, training, and workshops, practitioners can enable individuals in the community to take an active role in their own healthcare, thus promoting resilience, agency, and self-sufficiency. Herbal medicine can also assist in creating networks of support, solidarity, and mutual aid within communities, enabling them to address their healthcare needs and challenges jointly. This is achieved by encouraging collaboration and partnership between local healers, herbalists, healthcare providers, and community leaders.

To sum up, herbal medicine provides valuable answers to healthcare problems in environments with limited resources. It gives communities without access to traditional medical care accessible, reasonably priced, culturally appropriate, and long-lasting healthcare options. Herbal medicine has the potential to improve health outcomes, lessen health disparities, and increase resilience in environments with limited resources by utilizing the therapeutic potential of medicinal plants, fusing traditional healing methods with contemporary healthcare techniques, and encouraging community empowerment and self-reliance. Communities may use plant healing to create healthier, more resilient, and more equitable societies for future generations if they continue to support and invest in herbal medicine education, research, and infrastructure.

CONCLUSION

To sum up, "Herbal Solutions for Viral Challenges: A Journey Through Herbal Antiviral Practices" is a testament to the great promise that herbal therapy has when it comes to treating the intricate and constantly changing viral infection landscape. Readers have been immersed in a realm where contemporary science and old wisdom collide, providing a comprehensive strategy for effectively and resiliently addressing pandemic issues along this eye-opening trip.

The knowledge of ancient healing methods provides us with direction as we traverse the uncertainties of the contemporary world, showing us the road to a state of health and well-being based on the abundance of nature. Readers now possess a more profound comprehension of the bioactive chemicals, therapeutic mechanisms, and evidence-based methods that support the effectiveness of medicinal plants in fighting viruses, thanks to their investigation of herbal antiviral capabilities.

This trip has also shown how crucial it is for traditional herbal remedies and mainstream healthcare systems to work together and integrate. We can utilize the synergistic potential of herbal treatments to improve public health, promote wellness, and address the underlying causes of viral infections by bridging the gap between traditional wisdom and also contemporary research.

Upon contemplating the understandings and information obtained from this investigation, it is evident that the potency of herbal medicine is not limited to physical healing but also encompasses its potential to satiate the soul and promote adaptability in societies. Herbal medicine can be sustained as an essential resource for future generations by cultivating sustainable practices, ethical sourcing, and cultural preservation.

"Herbal Solutions for Viral Challenges" is a ray of hope and empowerment in the face of persistent viral threats and global health issues, encouraging readers to embrace nature's healing potential and set out on their own path to holistic wellbeing. We can successfully negotiate the complexity of viral issues by respecting the knowledge of the past and seizing the opportunities of the future.

Thank you for buying and reading/ listening to our book. If you found this book useful/ helpful please take a few minutes and leave a review on the platform where you purchased our book. Your feedback matters greatly to us.